To our very dear children and grandchildren

# Table of Contents

Chapter 1: Common Single Herbs — 5
Chapter 2: Herbs for Gastrointestinal System — 11
Chapter 3: Herbs for Musculoskeletal System — 17
Chapter 4: Herbs for Cardiovascular/Renal System — 23
Chapter 5: Herbs for Respiratory System — 29
Chapter 6: Herbs for Articular System — 35
Chapter 7: Herbs for Endocrine/Reproductive System — 41
Chapter 8: Herbs for Hematologic/Immunologic System — 47
Chapter 9: Herbs for Skin — 53
Chapter 10: Herbs for Nervous System — 59
Chapter 11: Herbs that Detoxify — 65
Chapter 12: Herbs for Emotional/Mental Well-being — 71
Crossword Puzzle Answer Keys — 79
About the Authors — 93

# Medical Disclaimer

You should always consult your licensed healthcare practitioner before making any changes to your medications, supplements, exercise, and diet. The information provided in this book is intended for educational purposes and should not be used as a substitute for professional medical advice. Collecting and interpreting your medical history should be approached with caution if you are not a licensed health professional. It is essential to collaborate with licensed healthcare providers to ensure the safety and appropriateness of any recommended Ayurvedic treatments.

# Welcome to a World of Healing Wisdom and Puzzle Adventures!

Thank you for picking up Holistic Healing with Herbs: Herbal Wisdom and Puzzle Adventures for Healing and Vitality, a book crafted to ignite your curiosity and deepen your appreciation for nature's gifts. Here, ancient herbal knowledge meets the thrill of brain-teasing puzzles, offering a unique blend of learning and entertainment.

Ayurveda, the "Science of Life," has cherished the healing power of herbs for thousands of years. Now, you can explore this time-honored wisdom in a playful, engaging way. Each puzzle invites you to uncover the names, uses, and benefits of various herbs, expanding your understanding and making your journey with Ayurveda both fun and meaningful.

Whether you're an avid student of natural medicine, a wellness enthusiast, or someone who loves a good challenge, We hope these pages bring you joy, insight, and a renewed connection to the healing secrets of the earth.

Happy puzzling, and may this adventure be as enlightening as it is enjoyable!

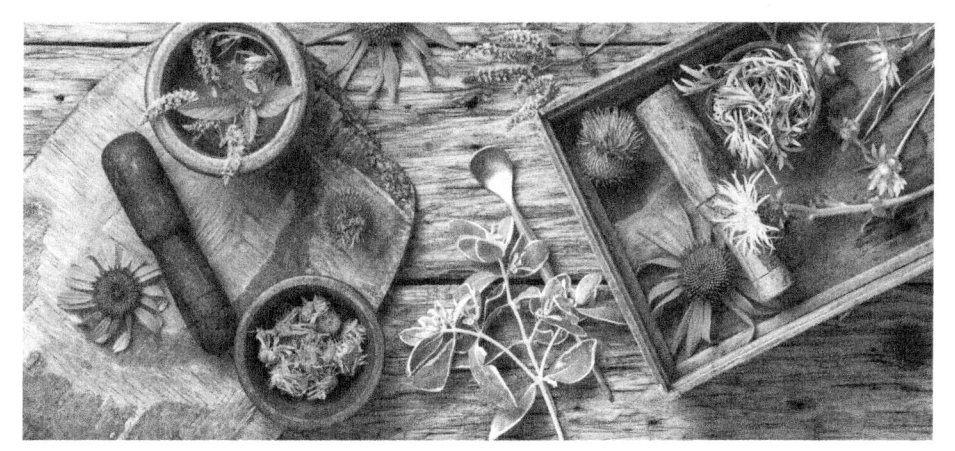

## Chapter 1
# Common Single Herbs

**Amalaki**: Amalaki is a highly nutritive herb known for its rejuvenative properties that support the health of the Dhatus (tissues). It is particularly beneficial for improving digestion and is widely used in the treatment of liver diseases and various skin problems due to its detoxifying and antioxidant effects.

**Ashwagandha**: Renowned for boosting strength, stamina, and immunity, Ashwagandha is a powerful adaptogen that helps manage stress and anxiety. It is also useful in alleviating nerve pain and supporting overall vitality, making it a staple in Ayurvedic therapies aimed at restoring balance and vigor.

**Bala**: Bala is an excellent tonic for strengthening the Dhatus, especially beneficial in cases of debility and undernourishment. It enhances physical resilience and promotes muscle health, making it a valuable herb for restoring energy and supporting healthy weight maintenance.

**Bibhitaki**: Bibhitaki is commonly used for relieving cough and congestion, helping clear the respiratory pathways. Additionally, it is recognized for its ability to improve body tone and support the overall structural integrity of the body.

# Common Single Herbs

**Brahmi:** Brahmi is a calming herb that soothes the mind and enhances memory. It is frequently used to manage anxiety and pain, providing cognitive support while reducing mental fatigue and promoting a peaceful state of mind.

**Eranda:** Known for its strong purgative action, Eranda is used in Virechana (therapeutic purgation) and is effective in cleansing the body of toxins. It is also applied topically to relieve joint and abdominal pain, demonstrating its versatility in both internal and external use.

**Ginger:** Ginger is a warming herb that aids digestion, relieves nausea, and purifies the blood. It can also be applied topically to alleviate headaches and soothe aching joints, making it a highly valued remedy in traditional and modern medicine.

**Guduchi**: Guduchi is celebrated for its ability to strengthen digestion and is often used to treat hyperacidity, inflammation, and various skin conditions. It supports the immune system and is revered for its detoxifying and rejuvenating qualities.

**Guggulu**: Guggulu is a potent anti-inflammatory herb that benefits the joints and muscles, offering significant support in managing arthritis and muscular pain. It also serves as a detoxifier, helping to eliminate impurities from the body and improve overall vitality.

**Haritaki:** Haritaki is known for its cleansing and rejuvenative effects on the Dhatus, making it useful for maintaining digestive health and supporting the nervous system. It is especially effective for individuals experiencing weakness or nervous exhaustion.

# Common Single Herbs

**Katuka:** Katuka is a liver-cleansing herb that helps relieve constipation and nourishes the heart. It is also known for enhancing Agni (digestive fire), making it useful for improving digestive efficiency and overall metabolism.

**Kumari:** Kumari, or Aloe Vera, is widely used for its cooling properties that benefit the skin, treat anemia, and address various gynecological issues. It also helps to reduce excess heat in the body, making it an essential herb for balancing Pitta.

**Manjistha**: Manjistha is a blood purifier that enhances circulation and reduces inflammation. It is frequently used to support skin healing and is effective in treating skin conditions like acne, rashes, and other inflammatory disorders.

**Nagarmotha**: Nagarmotha is an herb that aids digestion and is often used to treat diarrhea. It is also applied topically to soothe itchy skin, demonstrating its dual role in promoting digestive and skin health.

**Neem**: Neem is a powerful detoxifying herb used to manage skin conditions, diabetes, and liver disorders. It is also highly effective in cleansing and disinfecting wounds, owing to its strong antibacterial and anti-inflammatory properties.

**Pippali**: Pippali strengthens the lungs and acts as an expectorant, making it useful for conditions like bronchitis, cough, and asthma. It enhances respiratory function and supports the body's natural defense mechanisms.

# Common Single Herbs

**Punarnava:** Punarnava is known for reducing swelling and supporting urinary health. It also benefits liver function, making it a key herb in detoxification and in the management of fluid retention and related conditions.

**Shatavari:** Shatavari is revered for promoting reproductive health and increasing Ojas (vital energy). It is commonly used to soothe ulcers and manage hyperacidity, providing nourishment and support to the female reproductive system.

**Tulsi**: Tulsi, or Holy Basil, is a revered herb that supports respiratory health and has strong antibacterial properties. It is often used to alleviate coughs and colds, offering protection and relief from respiratory infections.

**Yashtimadhu**: Yashtimadhu, or Licorice, is known for soothing the throat and helping with ulcers. It is also used to support respiratory and digestive health, providing a calming and protective effect on mucous membranes.

# Give your brain a workout and put your knowledge to the test with the following engaging crossword puzzle!

Complete the crossword on the next pages or online at AyurvedaPartner.com/HolisticHealingWithHerbs.html.

# Common Single Herbs

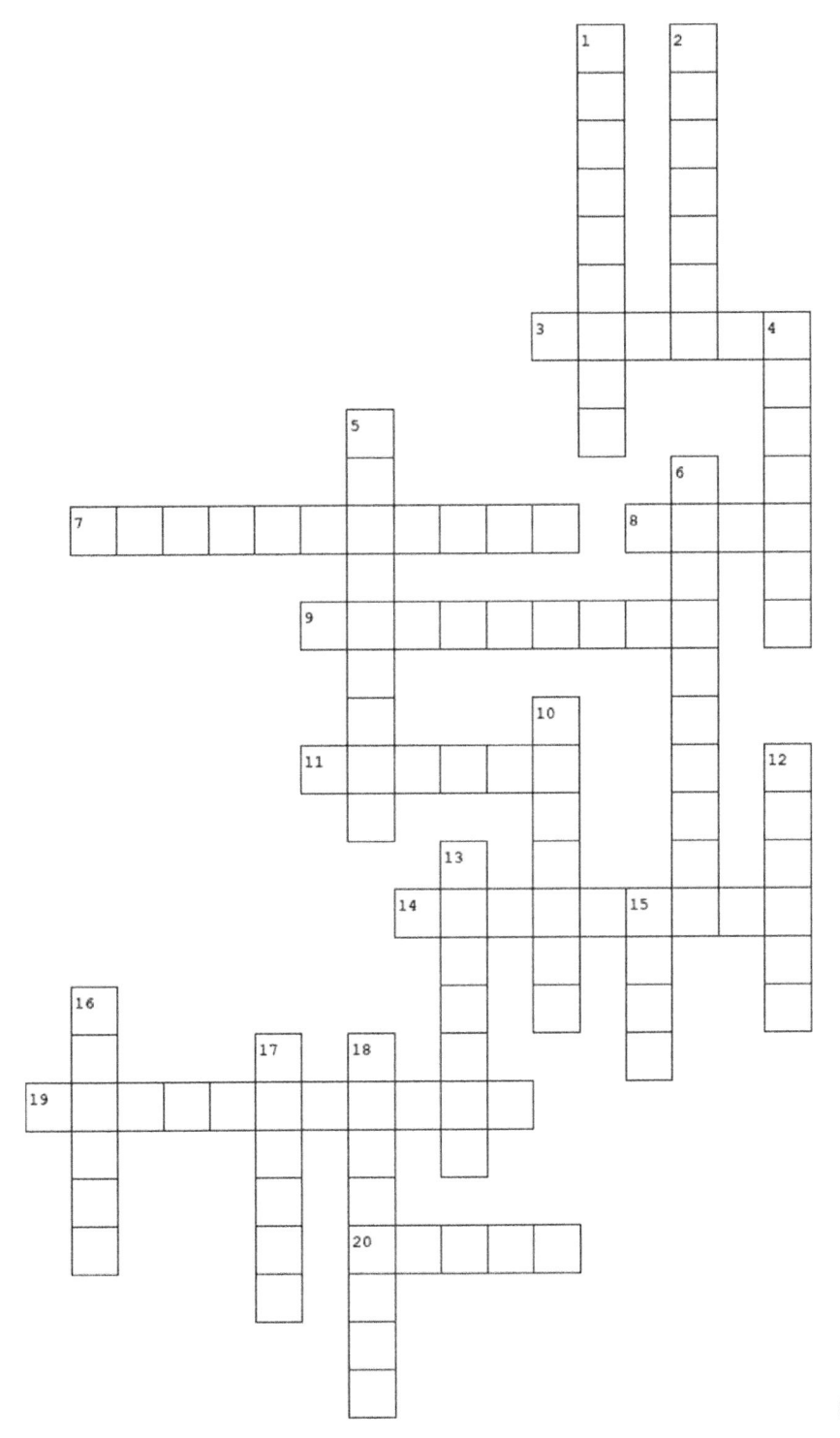

# Common Single Herbs

## Across

3. Cleanses liver, used for constipation, nourishes heart, improves Agni

7. Improves strength, stamina, immunity, helps with stress, anxiety, nerve pain

8. Strengthens Dhatus, useful in debility and undernourishment

9. Purifies blood, improves circulation, reduces inflammation, helps skin healing

11. Calms mind, enhances memory, helps with anxiety and pain

14. Reduces swelling, supports urinary health, helps with liver function

19. Soothes throat, helps with ulcers, used for respiratory and digestive health

20. Supports respiratory health, antibacterial, used in coughs and colds.

## Down

1. Used for cough, congestion, and improving body tone.

2. Anti-inflammatory, good for joints and muscles, detoxifies.

4. Nutritive, rejuvenates Dhatus, good for digestion, used in liver diseases and skin problems.

5. Promotes reproductive health, increases Ojas, used for ulcers, hyperacidity.

6. Aids digestion, used for diarrhea, applied to itchy skin.

10. Strengthens lungs, expectorant, used for bronchitis, cough, asthma.

12. Used for skin, anemia, gynecological issues, reduces heat.

13. Strengthens digestion, used in hyperacidity, inflammation, and skin conditions.

15. Used in skin conditions, diabetes, liver issues, cleanses wounds.

16. Strong purgative, used for Virechana, topical use for joints and abdomen.

17. Aids digestion, relieves nausea, purifies blood, topical use for headaches and joints.

18. Cleanses Dhatus, rejuvenates, useful for nervous system weakness and digestion.

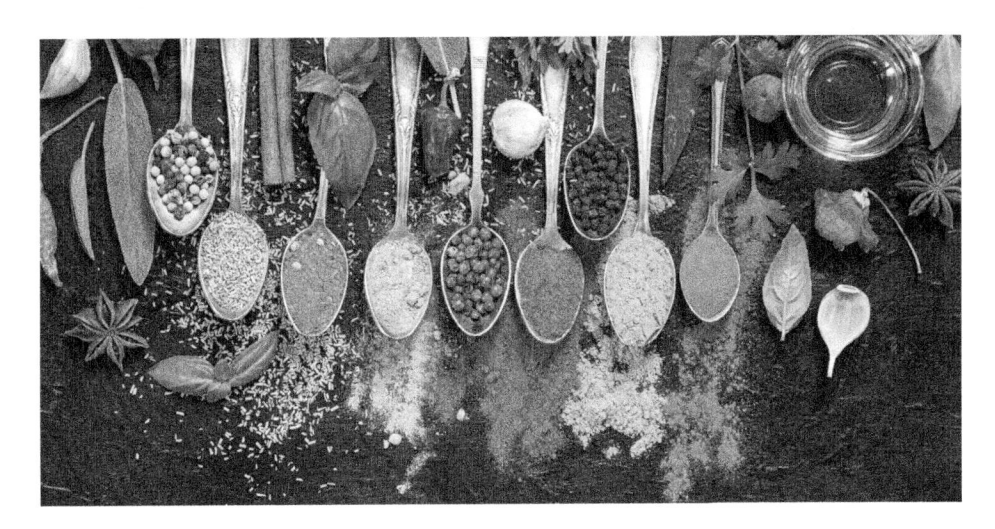

## Chapter 2
# Herbs for the Gastrointestinal System

**Ajwain:** Ajwain, also known as carom seeds, is a potent digestive aid used to relieve indigestion. Its active compounds work to accelerate the digestive process and reduce gas formation, providing quick relief from stomach pain, bloating, and discomfort caused by overeating.

**Amla:** Amla, a rejuvenating fruit high in Vitamin C, is great for gut health. It enhances digestion by stimulating gastric juices, balances stomach acid, and cleanses the intestines. Amla's high antioxidant content also rejuvenates the digestive tract and supports regular bowel movements.

**Avipattikar** Churna: Avipattikar Churna is a herbal formula used to manage hyperacidity and indigestion. It soothes excess stomach acid, promotes the smooth passage of food, and alleviates digestive discomfort, making it a powerful remedy for those suffering from acid reflux or gastric irritation.

**Bibhitaki**: Bibhitaki is one of the three fruits in Triphala and is highly beneficial for digestion. It tones the digestive tract, helps eliminate excess mucus, and supports proper elimination, making it ideal for those with irregular bowel movements or respiratory congestion.

# Herbs for the Gastrointestinal System

**Coriander:** Coriander seeds are highly effective in cooling excess heat in the stomach and supporting digestion. This cooling herb helps balance Pitta dosha, soothes inflammation, and promotes healthy digestive enzyme activity, making it ideal for those with a sensitive or overactive digestive system.

**Cumin:** Cumin is a common spice cherished for its ability to promote digestion and metabolism. It stimulates the secretion of digestive enzymes, which helps in breaking down food efficiently and reducing bloating. Cumin's warming properties also make it a favorite for soothing the digestive system and supporting gut health.

**Dashamula:** Dashamula, a blend of ten roots, is traditionally used to strengthen the digestive system. It has anti-inflammatory and detoxifying properties that improve digestion, reduce abdominal bloating, and support the body's natural ability to process and eliminate waste effectively.

**Fennel:** Fennel seeds are known for soothing the digestive system and reducing bloating. They have antispasmodic properties that relax the muscles of the gastrointestinal tract, making them effective in relieving stomach cramps, indigestion, and promoting overall digestive comfort.

**Ginger:** Ginger is a warming herb widely used to boost digestion and reduce nausea. Its stimulating nature increases digestive fire (Agni) and helps break down proteins more efficiently, while also reducing feelings of bloating and discomfort. It's particularly useful for people experiencing sluggish digestion or motion sickness.

# Herbs for the Gastrointestinal System

**Guduchi:** Guduchi is an immune-boosting herb that aids liver function, playing a vital role in supporting digestion. It helps to balance the gut microbiome, reduce inflammation, and improve the body's ability to break down and assimilate nutrients, making it beneficial for overall digestive health.

**Haritaki:** Haritaki, often referred to as the "King of Herbs," is known for aiding in bowel cleansing. It enhances digestion by removing toxins and supporting healthy elimination, while also nourishing the gut and strengthening the digestive system.

**Hing:** Hing, also known as Asafoetida, is a strong-smelling spice used to combat bloating and gas. It works by reducing spasms and improving the flow of digestive juices, making it a powerful remedy for flatulence, constipation, and sluggish digestion.

**Hingvastak Churna:** Hingvastak Churna is a compound remedy known for balancing Vata and easing bloating. This blend of spices and herbs, including asafoetida, enhances digestive fire and helps eliminate gas, making it an excellent choice for those with weak digestion or chronic bloating issues.

**Kutki:** Kutki is a bitter herb that supports liver and digestive health. It stimulates bile flow, aiding in the efficient digestion of fats, and has detoxifying effects on the liver, making it an excellent herb for cleansing and enhancing metabolic function.

**Licorice:** Licorice is renowned for soothing and protecting the stomach lining. Its mucilaginous properties form a protective layer over the stomach walls, reducing irritation and promoting healing in cases of ulcers and gastritis, while also supporting overall digestive comfort.

# Herbs for the Gastrointestinal System

**Musta:** Musta is commonly used for easing stomach discomfort and diarrhea. Its antispasmodic and anti-inflammatory properties calm the intestines, relieve digestive distress, and help restore balance to the digestive system, especially in cases of excess Pitta or Kapha.

**Pippali:** Pippali, an Ayurvedic pepper, enhances digestive fire and helps in the proper absorption of nutrients. It is especially effective for respiratory and digestive health, stimulating metabolism and alleviating issues like indigestion, gas, and sluggish digestion.

**Shatavari:** Shatavari is a cooling herb that helps with gastric ulcers and supports healthy digestion. Its soothing and anti-inflammatory properties protect the stomach lining and promote the secretion of digestive enzymes, making it particularly useful for individuals with hyperacidity or sensitive stomachs.

**Triphala:** Triphala is a powerful blend of three fruits (Amalaki, Bibhitaki, and Haritaki) used for digestive health. It gently cleanses the digestive tract, promotes regular bowel movements, and supports the assimilation of nutrients, making it an essential remedy for maintaining overall gut wellness.

# Get ready to challenge your mind and have fun as you tackle this exciting crossword puzzle!

Complete the crossword on the next pages or online at AyurvedaPartner.com/HolisticHealingWithHerbs.html.

# Herbs for the Gastrointestinal System

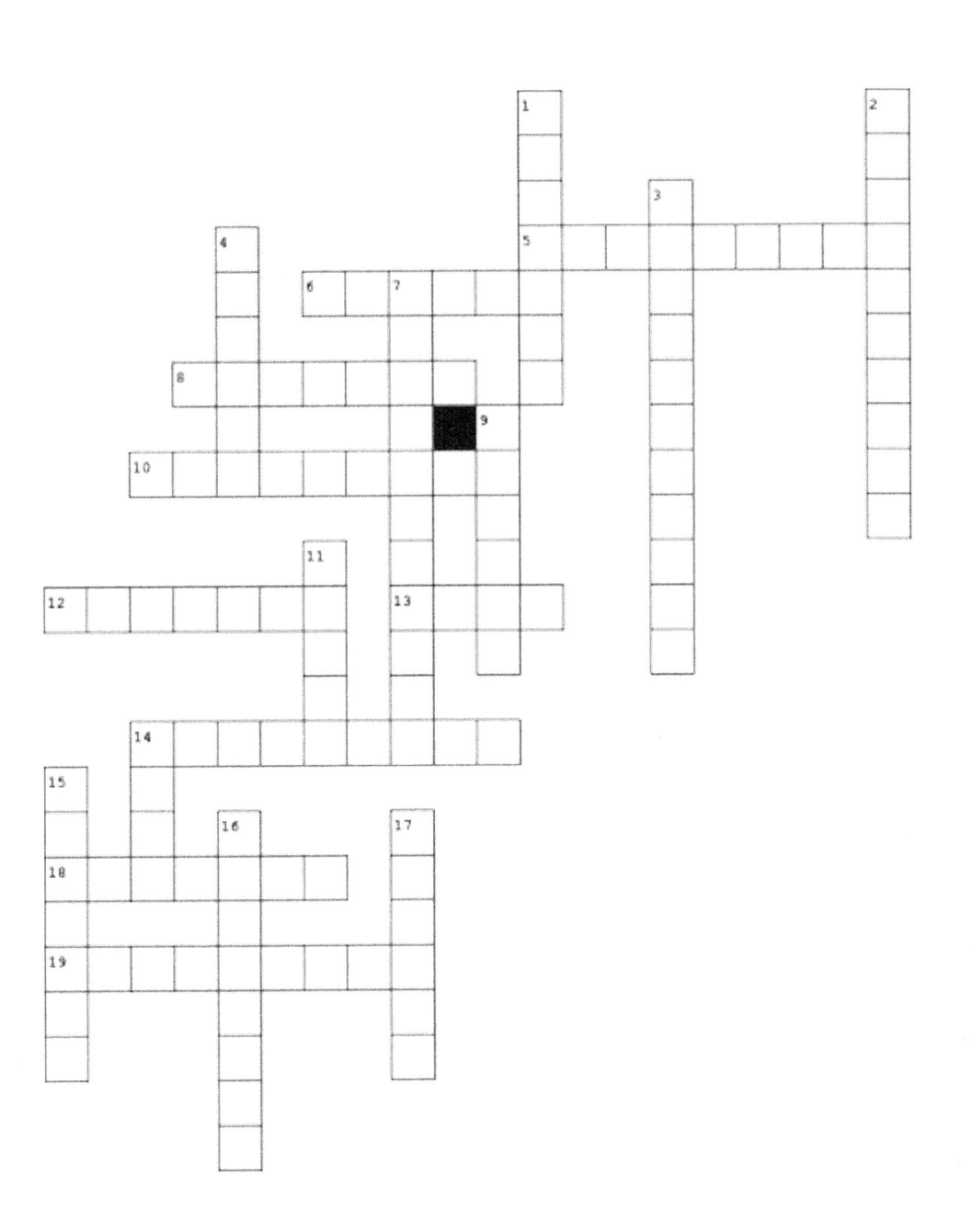

15

# Herbs for the Gastrointestinal System

## Across

3. A herbal formula used for hyperacidity and indigestion (two words)
5. Known as the "King of Herbs" and aids in bowel cleansing
7. Used for easing stomach discomfort and diarrhea
10. A blend of ten roots used to strengthen the digestive system
12. A compound remedy for balancing Vata and easing bloating (two words)
17. A warming herb often used to boost digestion and reduce nausea
18. A bitter herb that supports liver and digestive health
19. Cools excess heat in the stomach and supports digestion
20. Soothes and protects the stomach lining

## Down

1. A cooling herb that helps with gastric ulcers and digestion
2. An Ayurvedic pepper that enhances digestive fire
4. A powerful blend of three fruits for digestive health
6. A rejuvenating fruit high in Vitamin C, great for gut health
8. Also known as carom seeds, used to relieve indigestion
9. One of the three fruits in Triphala, great for digestion
11. A common spice used to promote digestion and metabolism
13. Rich in Vitamin C and rejuvenates the digestive tract
14. Also known as Asafoetida, used to combat bloating and gas
15. An immune-boosting herb that aids liver function
16. Soothes the digestive system and reduces bloating

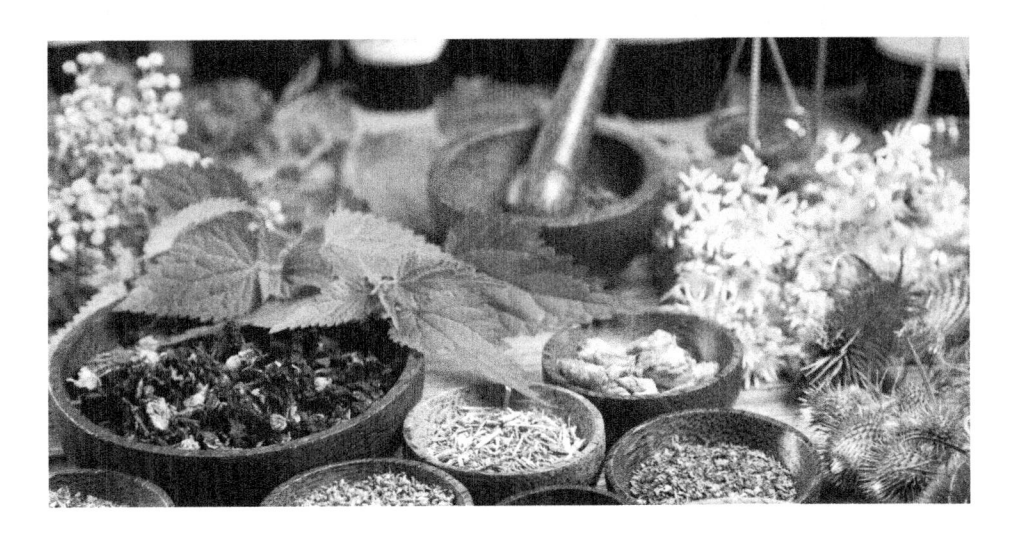

# Chapter 3
# Herbs for the Musculoskeletal System

**Amalaki:** Amalaki is known for providing antioxidant support, which plays a crucial role in tissue repair and bone health. It helps reduce oxidative stress in the musculoskeletal system, promoting recovery and overall resilience of bones and joints.

**Ashwagandha:** Ashwagandha is a revered herb that supports muscle strength and joint flexibility. It enhances the body's endurance and helps reduce inflammation, making it valuable for maintaining healthy, agile muscles and joints, especially under physical strain.

**Bala:** Bala is a potent herb that strengthens muscles and alleviates joint pain. It provides nourishment to the musculoskeletal system, enhancing muscle tone and supporting the recovery of connective tissues, which is beneficial for athletes and those with physical discomfort.

# Herbs for the Musculoskeletal System

**Bibhitaki:** Bibhitaki assists in maintaining joint health and fluidity. It helps lubricate the joints, improving mobility and reducing stiffness, making it useful for individuals dealing with joint discomfort or conditions like arthritis.

**Castor Oil:** Castor Oil is traditionally used to lubricate joints and reduce inflammation. Its natural properties soothe the musculoskeletal system, relieving joint pain and stiffness while promoting better joint function when applied topically.

**Guduchi:** Guduchi is a powerful herb that enhances tissue regeneration and reduces swelling. It supports the body's natural healing processes, promoting the recovery of muscles and joints and maintaining healthy connective tissue.

**Guggulu:** Guggulu is well-known for helping to reduce inflammation and maintain joint mobility. It supports the musculoskeletal system by protecting joints from stiffness and deterioration, aiding in the management of chronic pain and arthritis.

**Haritaki:** Haritaki is valued for improving flexibility and supporting musculoskeletal detoxification. It aids in eliminating toxins that can accumulate in the muscles and joints, enhancing overall fluidity and promoting healthy joint movement.

**Kapikacchu:** Kapikacchu supports muscle relaxation and joint stability. It nourishes the muscles and nerves, helping to reduce muscle tension and promoting balanced joint function, which is essential for physical activities and maintaining postural alignment.

# Herbs for the Musculoskeletal System

**Laksha:** Laksha is an effective herb for promoting bone healing and tissue regeneration. It is particularly useful for accelerating the repair of fractures and strengthening the skeletal structure, ensuring better recovery and resilience of bones.

**Mahanarayan Oil:** Mahanarayan Oil is used topically to soothe sore muscles and joints. Its therapeutic blend of herbs penetrates deeply into the tissues, relieving pain, improving circulation, and reducing inflammation, which is ideal for post-exercise recovery or chronic joint issues.

**Moringa:** Moringa is rich in calcium and vitamins that are essential for bone health. It fortifies the musculoskeletal system by promoting bone density and reducing the risk of osteoporosis, while also supporting muscle function with its nutrient-rich profile.

**Musta:** Musta is beneficial for reducing muscle inflammation and stiffness. It soothes muscle tissue and alleviates pain, making it effective in relieving musculoskeletal discomfort caused by overuse or chronic conditions.

**Nirgundi:** Nirgundi is known for relieving muscle spasms and joint discomfort. Its anti-inflammatory properties help ease pain and swelling, making it a go-to remedy for muscular and joint issues, especially in conditions like arthritis.

**Punarnava:** Punarnava helps reduce joint swelling and inflammation. It has natural diuretic properties that reduce water retention around joints, relieving discomfort and promoting better joint mobility.

# Herbs for the Musculoskeletal System

**Rasna:** Rasna is an herb well-known for relieving joint pain and promoting flexibility. It soothes irritated tissues and helps restore mobility, making it a staple in managing musculoskeletal disorders and improving range of motion.

**Sahachara:** Sahachara provides relief from muscular pain and joint stiffness. It supports the relaxation of tense muscles and promotes overall joint comfort, making it beneficial for chronic musculoskeletal issues or post-exercise recovery.

**Shallaki:** Shallaki is commonly used to promote joint health and alleviate pain. It contains natural compounds that reduce inflammation and protect cartilage, helping to maintain joint function and ease discomfort in conditions like osteoarthritis.

**Shatavari:** Shatavari nourishes and strengthens bones and connective tissues. Its rejuvenating properties support skeletal health, making it an excellent herb for improving bone density and enhancing the integrity of ligaments and tendons.

**Turmeric:** Turmeric is a powerful anti-inflammatory herb containing curcumin, which is known for its ability to alleviate joint pain and muscle soreness. It reduces inflammation throughout the musculoskeletal system, promoting long-term joint health and mobility.

## Ready to think? Dive into this thrilling crossword and test your mastery!

Complete the crossword on the next pages or online at AyurvedaPartner.com/HolisticHealingWithHerbs.html.

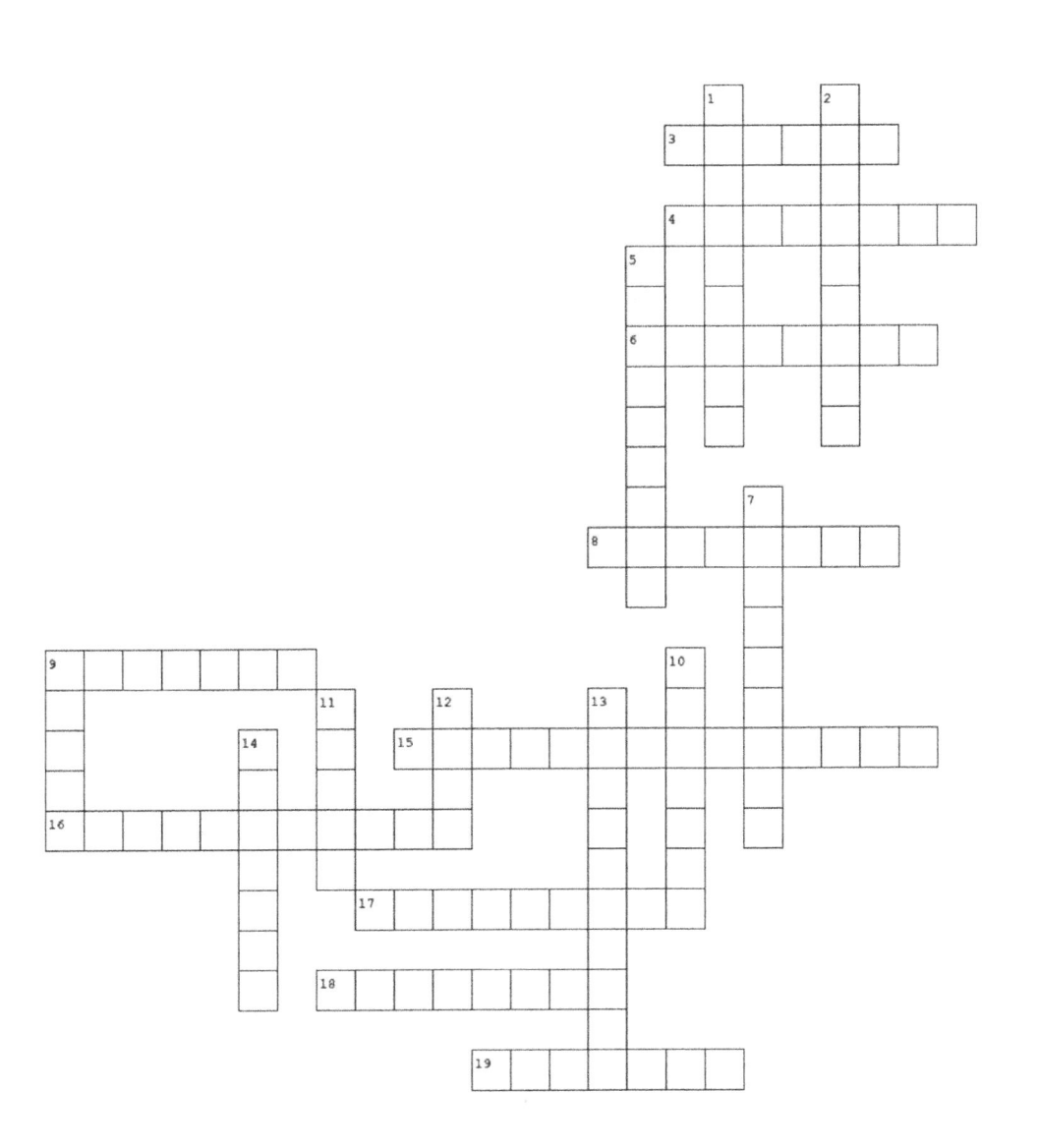

# Herbs for the Musculoskeletal System

# Herbs for the Musculoskeletal System

## Across

3. Promotes bone healing and tissue regeneration

4. Improves flexibility and supports musculoskeletal detoxification

6. Promotes joint health and alleviates pain

8. Relieves muscle spasms and joint discomfort

9. Rich in calcium and vitamins for bone health

15. Used topically to soothe sore muscles and joints (two words)

16. Supports muscle strength and joint flexibility

17. Assists in maintaining joint health and fluidity

18. Contains curcumin, known for its powerful anti-inflammatory properties

19. Enhances tissue regeneration and reduces swelling

## Down

1. Provides relief from muscular pain and joint stiffness

2. Nourishes and strengthens bones and connective tissues

5. Lubricates joints and helps reduce inflammation (two words

7. Helps reduce joint swelling and inflammation

9. Reduces muscle inflammation and stiffness

10. Provides antioxidant support for tissue repair and bone health

11. Known for relieving joint pain and promoting flexibility

12. Strengthens muscles and alleviates joint pain

13. Supports muscle relaxation and joint stability

14. Helps reduce inflammation and maintain joint mobility

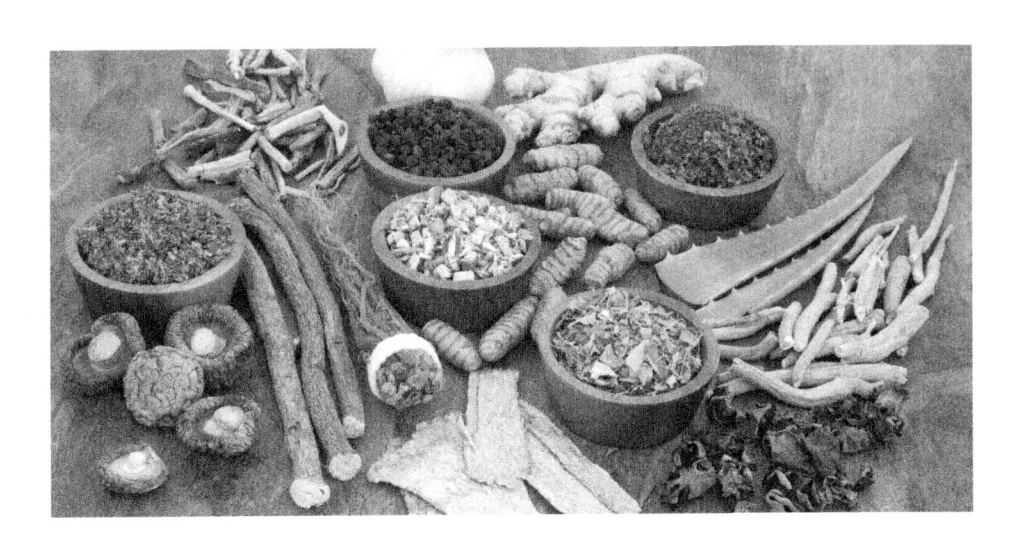

# Chapter 4
# Herbs for the Cardiovascular/Renal System

**Amla:** Amla, a rejuvenating fruit packed with Vitamin C, is vital for cardiovascular and renal health. It strengthens the heart by improving cardiac function and promotes kidney well-being by supporting detoxification processes, making it an essential herb for overall vitality.

**Arjuna:** Arjuna bark is a revered herb in Ayurveda for heart health, known for its ability to improve circulation and strengthen cardiac muscles. It helps maintain healthy blood pressure levels and supports the cardiovascular system, ensuring efficient blood flow and heart function.

**Ashwagandha:** Ashwagandha, an adaptogenic herb, is valued for its stress-relieving properties that positively impact heart health. By reducing cortisol levels, it supports cardiovascular function and helps the heart cope with daily stress, making it essential for heart health and emotional well-being.

# Herbs for the Cardiovascular/Renal System

**Bhumyamalaki:** Bhumyamalaki is a protective herb for the liver and kidneys, aiding in the detoxification of these crucial organs. It supports renal health by promoting efficient waste elimination and reducing the risk of kidney-related issues, making it a valuable herb for overall cleansing.

**Brahmi:** Brahmi is an herb that enhances cognitive function while also benefiting the cardiovascular system. It calms the mind, reduces stress, and supports healthy blood flow, promoting heart health and mental clarity simultaneously.

**Cinnamon:** Cinnamon is a warming spice that supports heart health by helping to lower blood sugar and cholesterol levels. It improves circulation, making it beneficial for cardiovascular wellness and ensuring that the heart and blood vessels remain in optimal condition.

**Coriander:** Coriander is a cooling herb that not only aids digestion but also supports kidney function. It promotes the excretion of excess fluids and helps detoxify the urinary system, making it an excellent herb for overall kidney health.

**Fennel:** Fennel seeds are known for their digestive benefits, but they also play a significant role in supporting urinary health. They act as a diuretic, helping to flush out toxins from the kidneys and maintaining a balanced fluid level in the body.

**Garlic:** Garlic is a powerful bulb known for its ability to reduce cholesterol levels and support heart health. Its active compounds help dilate blood vessels, lower blood pressure, and improve overall cardiovascular function, protecting against heart disease.

# Herbs for the Cardiovascular/Renal System

**Gokshura:** Gokshura is an herb highly regarded for promoting kidney and bladder function. It helps in the detoxification process, supports urinary tract health, and ensures the efficient elimination of waste from the body, contributing to overall renal wellness.

**Guduchi:** Guduchi is an immune-boosting herb that plays a crucial role in supporting kidney and liver function. It enhances the body's natural detoxification processes, reducing inflammation and promoting the efficient functioning of these vital organs.

**Hibiscus:** Hibiscus is a flower celebrated for its ability to lower blood pressure and improve heart function. It contains natural antioxidants that relax the blood vessels, promoting better circulation and supporting overall cardiovascular health.

**Manjistha:** Manjistha is a root known for purifying the blood and supporting the circulatory system. It detoxifies the blood, helps maintain healthy blood flow, and reduces inflammation, making it a crucial herb for circulatory well-being.

**Neem:** Neem is a powerful detoxifying herb used to purify the blood and improve circulation. It helps clear toxins from the bloodstream, supports heart health, and promotes overall vascular function, protecting the cardiovascular system from damage.

**Punarnava:** Punarnava is a rejuvenating herb that reduces swelling and supports kidney health. It acts as a natural diuretic, aiding in the elimination of excess fluids and preventing water retention, making it effective for maintaining kidney function and reducing inflammation.

# Herbs for the Cardiovascular/Renal System

**Shankhpushpi:** Shankhpushpi is a calming plant that benefits the cardiovascular system by reducing stress and anxiety. It supports heart health by lowering blood pressure and promoting a relaxed state, ensuring smooth blood flow and heart efficiency.

**Shatavari:** Shatavari is an adaptogenic herb that promotes hormonal balance and supports kidney function. It nourishes and protects the kidneys, helping to maintain fluid balance in the body and ensuring that the renal system operates smoothly.

**Triphala:** Triphala, a blend of three fruits, is a powerful formula known for its detoxifying properties. It supports renal health by cleansing the kidneys and promoting efficient waste elimination, ensuring that the body remains free of toxins and well-balanced.

**Tulsi:** Tulsi, also known as Holy Basil, is an herb used to lower stress and support cardiovascular well-being. It has adaptogenic properties that help balance cortisol levels, reduce inflammation, and promote healthy heart function, protecting the cardiovascular system.

**Turmeric:** Turmeric is a golden root rich in curcumin, known for its potent anti-inflammatory properties. It supports cardiovascular health by reducing inflammation in blood vessels, improving circulation, and protecting the heart from oxidative stress, ensuring overall well-being.

## Get ready to spark your mind with this exciting crossword—can you conquer it?

Complete the crossword on the next pages or online at AyurvedaPartner.com/HolisticHealingWithHerbs.html.

# Herbs for the Cardiovascular/Renal System

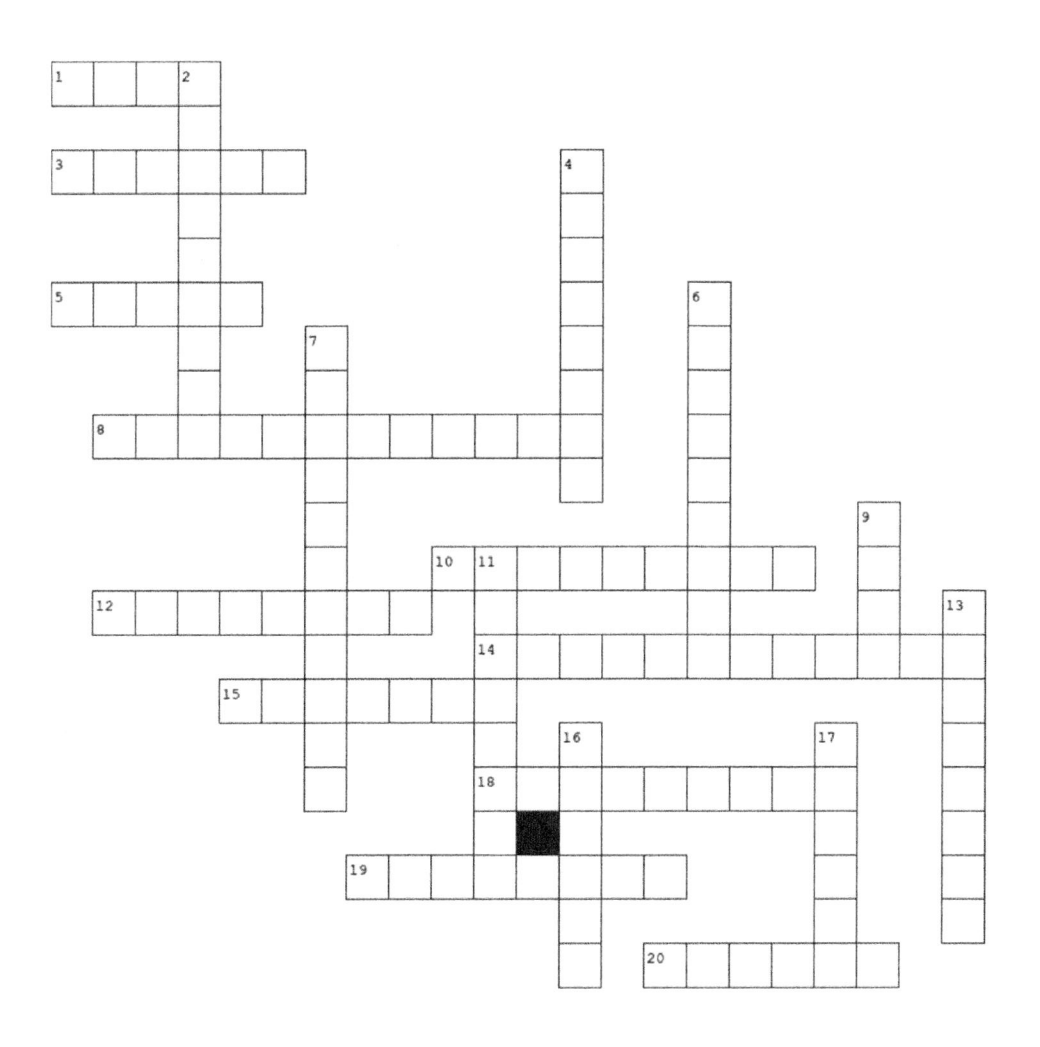

# Herbs for the Cardiovascular/Renal System

## Across

1. Powerful detoxifying herb for purifying the blood and improving circulation
3. Seed used to promote digestion and support urinary health
5. Herb used to lower stress and support cardiovascular well-being
8. Plant used to calm the mind and support cardiovascular health
10. Adaptogenic herb that promotes hormonal balance and kidney function
12. Blend of three fruits known for detoxification and supporting renal health
14. Herb known for protecting the liver and supporting renal health
15. Immune-boosting herb that supports kidney and liver function
18. Cooling herb used to promote digestion and support kidney function
19. Herb known for promoting kidney and bladder function
20. Bulb known for reducing cholesterol and supporting heart health

## Down

2. Root used to purify the blood and support the circulatory system
4. Root with anti-inflammatory properties that support cardiovascular health
6. A rejuvenating herb that helps reduce swelling and supports kidney health
7. Adaptogenic herb used to manage stress and improve heart function
9. Rejuvenating fruit that strengthens the heart and supports kidney health
11. Flower used to lower blood pressure and improve heart function
13. Warming spice that helps lower blood sugar and support heart health
16. Tree bark used to support heart health and improve circulation
17. Herb that improves cognitive function and benefits heart health

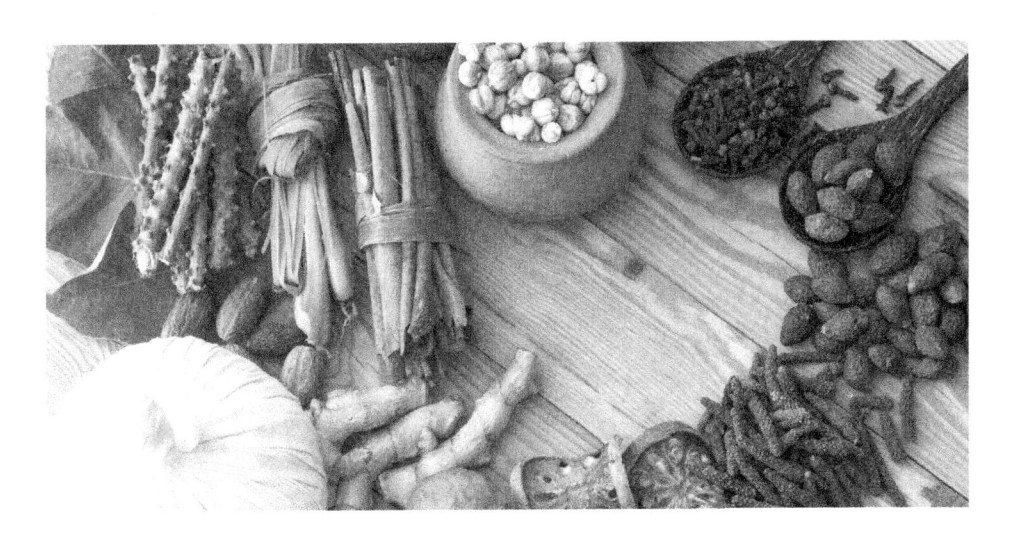

## Chapter 5
# Herbs for the Respiratory System

**Anantmool:** Anantmool is an essential herb for cleansing and supporting the respiratory channels. It helps to clear mucus and toxins from the lungs, promoting easy breathing and overall respiratory well-being, making it a great choice for lung detoxification.

**Bharangi:** Bharangi is known for alleviating respiratory congestion and soothing bronchial tissues. It helps open up airways, making it easier to breathe, and is often used to manage respiratory issues such as asthma and chronic bronchitis.

**Bay Leaf:** Bay Leaf is effective in reducing congestion and supporting breathing. Its aromatic properties help clear mucus from the respiratory tract, making it a natural remedy for colds and blocked sinuses, providing relief from respiratory discomfort.

**Camphor:** Camphor is used to clear respiratory passages and aid in easy breathing. Its strong, menthol-like aroma acts as a natural decongestant, making it a staple in treating colds, nasal congestion, and bronchial issues.

# Herbs for the Respiratory System

**Cardamom:** Cardamom is valued for clearing mucus and supporting healthy lung function. It has a warming effect on the respiratory system and helps in reducing phlegm buildup, making it useful for respiratory relief and promoting easy breathing.

**Cinnamon:** Cinnamon is a warming spice that supports the respiratory system by reducing mucus buildup. It helps to open up airways and soothe inflammation, making it ideal for managing colds, flu, and respiratory congestion.

**Clove:** Clove supports respiratory function and provides relief from cough. Its expectorant properties help clear mucus from the lungs and soothe the throat, making it an effective remedy for colds and respiratory infections.

**Eucalyptus Oil:** Eucalyptus Oil is well-known for clearing airways and relieving sinus congestion. Its strong, minty aroma helps to open nasal passages, providing immediate relief from stuffiness and promoting clearer breathing.

**Ginger:** Ginger is a powerful herb that reduces respiratory congestion and promotes lung health. It helps to break down and eliminate mucus, soothe the airways, and reduce inflammation in the respiratory system, making it ideal for respiratory relief.

**Haridra:** Haridra, also known as Turmeric, has strong anti-inflammatory properties that support lung health. It helps reduce inflammation in the respiratory system and provides relief from asthma and other bronchial conditions, promoting easier breathing.

# Herbs for the Respiratory System

**Holy Basil:** Holy Basil, known for its anti-inflammatory and immune-boosting effects, is a powerhouse for respiratory health. It helps reduce mucus buildup, clears the airways, and supports overall lung function, making it a key herb in managing respiratory infections.

**Kantakari:** Kantakari is used to reduce respiratory discomfort and soothe bronchial tissues. It helps clear mucus from the lungs and supports smooth, unobstructed breathing, making it beneficial for conditions like bronchitis and asthma.

**Neem:** Neem is a purifying herb that helps cleanse the respiratory system and alleviate respiratory infections. It has natural antibacterial and anti-inflammatory properties that aid in clearing the lungs and supporting immune defense.

**Pippali:** Pippali enhances lung function and reduces congestion. It is known for stimulating mucus clearance from the respiratory tract and supporting efficient lung function, making it helpful for those with chronic cough and respiratory distress.

**Pushkarmool:** Pushkarmool is a strengthening herb for the respiratory system, known for alleviating asthma symptoms. It helps to open up the airways, reduce inflammation, and promote better lung function, making breathing easier for those with respiratory conditions.

**Shirish:** Shirish is effective in reducing respiratory allergies and clearing lung channels. It helps alleviate symptoms of asthma and allergic bronchitis by purging toxins and soothing inflamed tissues, promoting better respiratory health.

# Herbs for the Respiratory System

**Trikatu:** Trikatu, a combination of three powerful spices, is used to clear mucus and boost respiratory function. It warms the body, stimulates circulation, and helps break down mucus buildup, making it ideal for clearing the respiratory tract and enhancing lung health.

**Tulsi:** Tulsi, also known as Holy Basil, is a potent herb for respiratory health that helps clear mucus from the lungs. It boosts the immune system, reduces inflammation, and opens up the airways, making it a must-have for respiratory wellness.

**Turmeric:** Turmeric is renowned for its anti-inflammatory properties that support lung health. It helps soothe the respiratory tract, reduce inflammation, and relieve symptoms of asthma and bronchial infections, making it a key herb for respiratory care.

**Vasaka:** Vasaka is a soothing herb that supports the respiratory tract and relieves bronchial conditions. It helps to reduce inflammation, open airways, and promote easier breathing, making it especially effective for chronic respiratory ailments.

## Prepare to ignite your curiosity and tackle this thrilling crossword puzzle—are you up for the ultimate brain-teasing adventure?

Complete the crossword on the next pages or online at AyurvedaPartner.com/HolisticHealingWithHerbs.html.

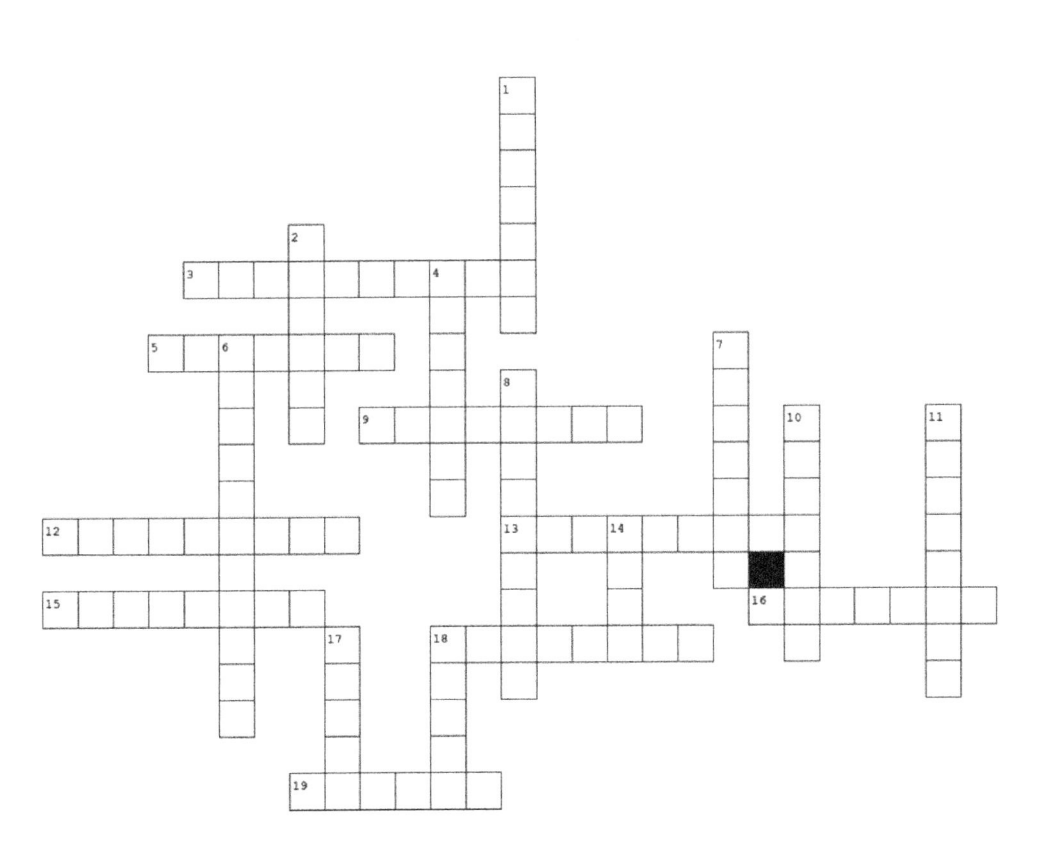

# Herbs for the Respiratory System

# Herbs for the Respiratory System

**Across**

3. Oil Clears airways and relieves sinus congestion

5. Enhances lung function and reduces congestion

9. Alleviates respiratory congestion and soothes bronchial tissues

12. Known for its anti-inflammatory and immune-boosting effects on the respiratory system (Two words)

13. Cleanses and supports the respiratory channels

15. Warms the respiratory system and reduces mucus build-up

16. Supports lung health and alleviates respiratory inflammation

18. Clears mucus and supports healthy lung function

19. Reduces respiratory congestion and promotes lung health

**Down**

1. Reduces respiratory allergies and clears lung channels

2. Soothes the respiratory tract and relieves bronchial conditions

4. A combination that helps clear mucus and boost respiratory function

6. Strengthens the respiratory system and alleviates asthma symptoms

7. Clears respiratory passages and helps with easy breathing

8. Reduces respiratory discomfort and soothes bronchial tissues

10. Helps reduce congestion and supports breathing (Two words)

11. Anti-inflammatory properties that support lung health

14. Purifies the respiratory system and alleviates respiratory infections

17. Supports respiratory health and helps clear mucus from the lungs

18. Supports respiratory function and helps with cough relief

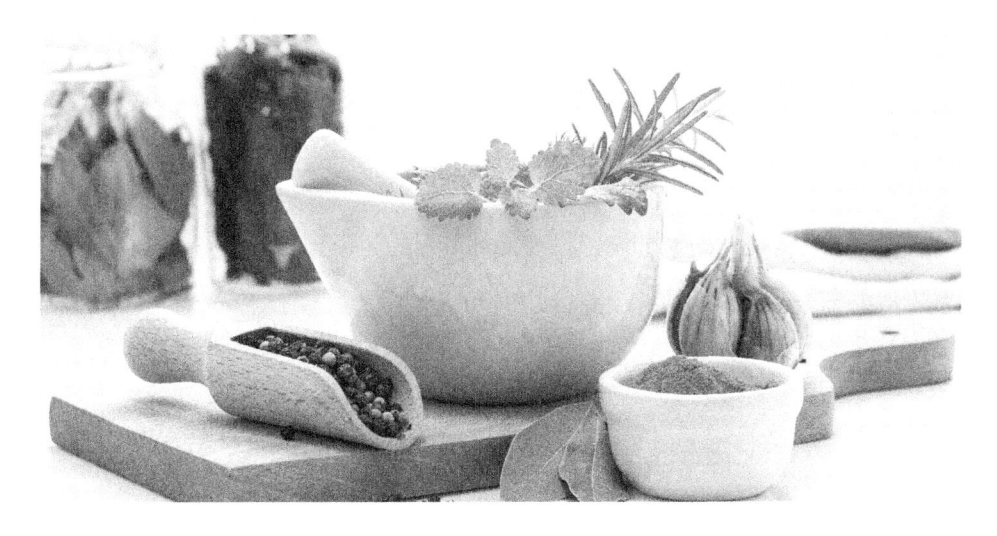

## Chapter 6
# Herbs for the Articular System

**Amalaki:** Amalaki provides powerful antioxidants that maintain joint function and support overall articular health. By reducing oxidative stress, it helps protect cartilage from degeneration and ensures smooth joint movement, making it an effective herb for long-term joint maintenance.

**Ashwagandha:** Ashwagandha is a rejuvenating herb that strengthens joints and helps reduce inflammation. It promotes the health of connective tissues and minimizes pain and swelling, making it valuable for individuals experiencing joint stiffness or arthritis.

**Bala:** Bala is renowned for strengthening joints and connective tissues. It nourishes the ligaments and tendons, enhancing their resilience and providing support to the articular system, which is essential for maintaining joint stability and flexibility.

**Castor Oil:** Castor Oil is used topically to lubricate joints and alleviate pain. Its anti-inflammatory properties penetrate deeply into the tissues, reducing swelling and stiffness, and providing relief for conditions such as arthritis and joint discomfort.

# Herbs for the Articular System

**Devadaru:** Devadaru is known for relieving joint stiffness and supporting joint mobility. It has anti-inflammatory and pain-relieving properties that make it effective for easing discomfort in conditions like osteoarthritis and rheumatoid arthritis.

**Guduchi:** Guduchi enhances joint health and reduces inflammatory conditions. It acts as a natural anti-inflammatory and immunomodulator, promoting the regeneration of joint tissues and supporting overall joint wellness.

**Guggulu:** Guggulu is highly effective in reducing swelling and promoting joint mobility. It helps detoxify the joints, reduces inflammation, and facilitates smoother movement, making it a key remedy for arthritis and joint stiffness.

**Haritaki:** Haritaki detoxifies the body and supports joint health by removing accumulated toxins that can contribute to inflammation. It enhances flexibility and protects joint tissues from damage, promoting overall joint wellness.

**Kapikacchu:** Kapikacchu promotes joint stability and muscle relaxation. It helps support the strength and flexibility of joints while easing muscle tension, making it beneficial for athletes and those experiencing joint discomfort.

**Khadira:** Khadira is a potent herb that helps reduce inflammation in the joints. It soothes swollen and irritated tissues, providing relief from pain and stiffness associated with chronic joint conditions.

# Herbs for the Articular System

**Laksha:** Laksha is known for promoting bone healing and joint regeneration. It supports the repair of damaged joint tissues and strengthens bones, making it a vital herb for recovering from fractures and joint injuries.

**Manjistha:** Manjistha purifies the blood and supports healthy joint function. By improving circulation and reducing inflammation, it ensures that nutrients reach the joints efficiently, promoting overall joint health and flexibility.

**Moringa:** Moringa is a nutrient-rich herb that provides essential vitamins and minerals to support joint and bone health. It helps reduce inflammation, nourish joint tissues, and improve overall articular function.

**Musta:** Musta is effective in reducing pain and swelling in inflamed joints. It acts as an anti-inflammatory agent, soothing joint discomfort and providing relief from arthritis and other inflammatory joint conditions.

**Nirgundi:** Nirgundi is known for relieving joint pain and muscle stiffness. Its anti-inflammatory and analgesic properties make it ideal for reducing swelling and improving mobility, ensuring better joint health and function.

**Punarnava:** Punarnava is a rejuvenating herb that reduces joint swelling and stiffness. It helps eliminate excess fluid buildup in the joints, alleviating discomfort and improving flexibility, making it beneficial for conditions like arthritis.

# Herbs for the Articular System

**Rasna:** Rasna is commonly used to ease joint discomfort and improve flexibility. It reduces inflammation and soothes irritated joint tissues, helping to restore movement and alleviate pain in the articular system.

**Shallaki:** Shallaki supports joint flexibility and alleviates pain. It contains natural anti-inflammatory compounds that protect cartilage and improve joint function, making it effective for managing chronic joint pain and stiffness.

**Shatavari:** Shatavari nourishes bones and supports healthy joints. It helps maintain the strength and integrity of the articular system, ensuring better flexibility and reducing the risk of joint-related disorders.

**Turmeric:** Turmeric contains curcumin, which is well-known for its anti-inflammatory benefits for joints. It helps reduce joint pain and swelling, making it a valuable herb for managing arthritis and promoting overall joint health.

# Challenge your wits and dive into this captivating crossword puzzle—can you master the twists and turns ahead?

Complete the crossword on the next pages or online at AyurvedaPartner.com/HolisticHealingWithHerbs.html.

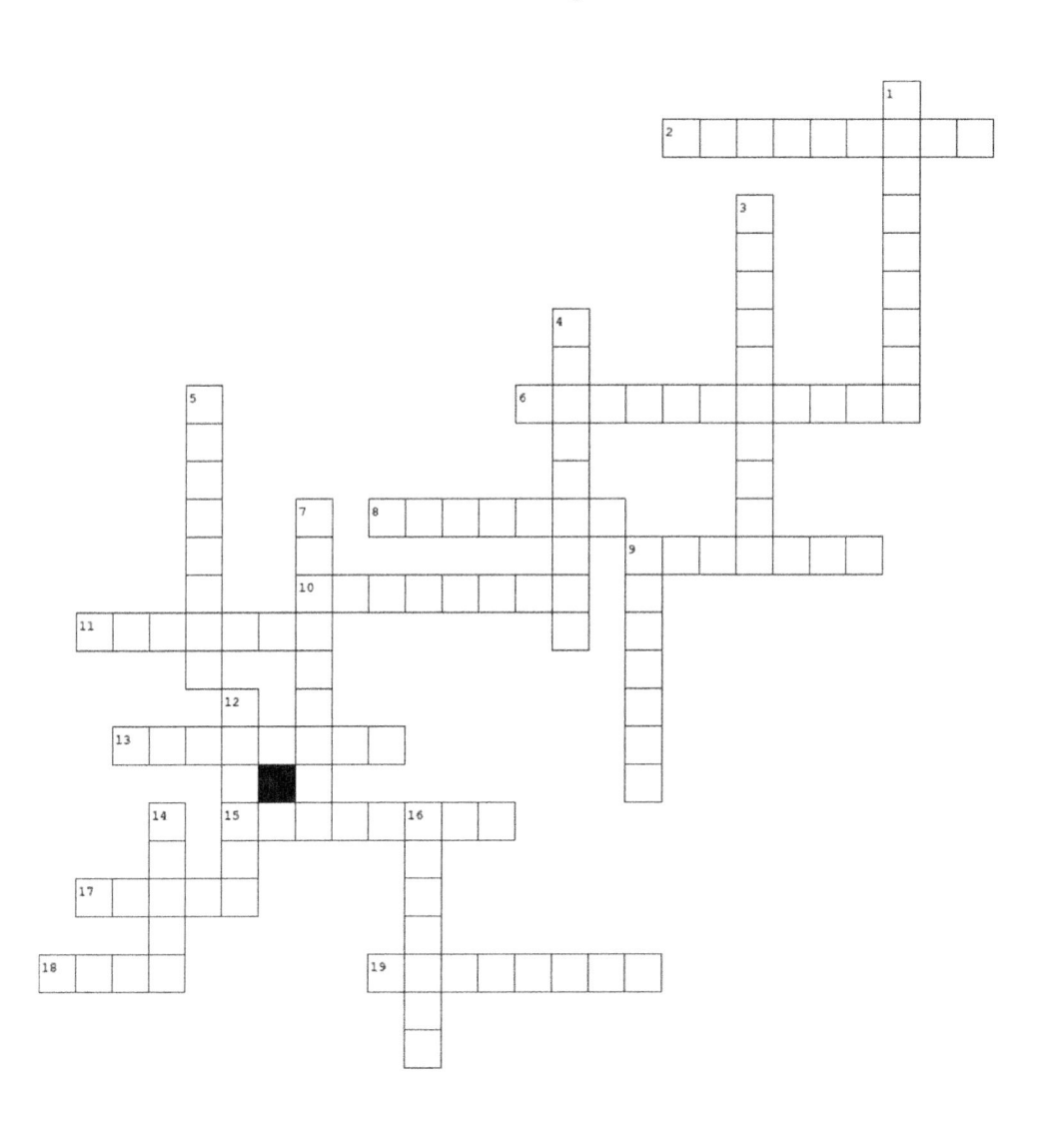

# Herbs for the Articular System

# Herbs for the Articular System

## Across

2. Nourishes bones and supports healthy joints

6. Strengthens joints and helps reduce inflammation

8. Helps reduce inflammation in the joints

9. Enhances joint health and reduces inflammatory conditions

10. Relieves joint pain and muscle stiffness

11. Provides nutrients that support joint and bone health

13. Relieves joint stiffness and supports joint mobility

15. Supports joint flexibility and alleviates pain

17. Reduces pain and swelling in inflamed joints

18. Strengthens joints and connective t issues

19. Detoxifies the body and supports joint health

## Down

1. Purifies the blood and supports healthy joint function

3. Promotes joint stability and muscle relaxation

4. Lubricates joints and alleviates pain when used topically (Two words)

5. Contains curcumin, known for its anti-inflammatory benefits for joints

7. Reduces joint swelling and stiffness

9. Reduces swelling and promotes joint mobility

12. Promotes bone healing and joint regeneration

14. Eases joint discomfort and improves flexibility

16. Provides antioxidants to maintain joint function

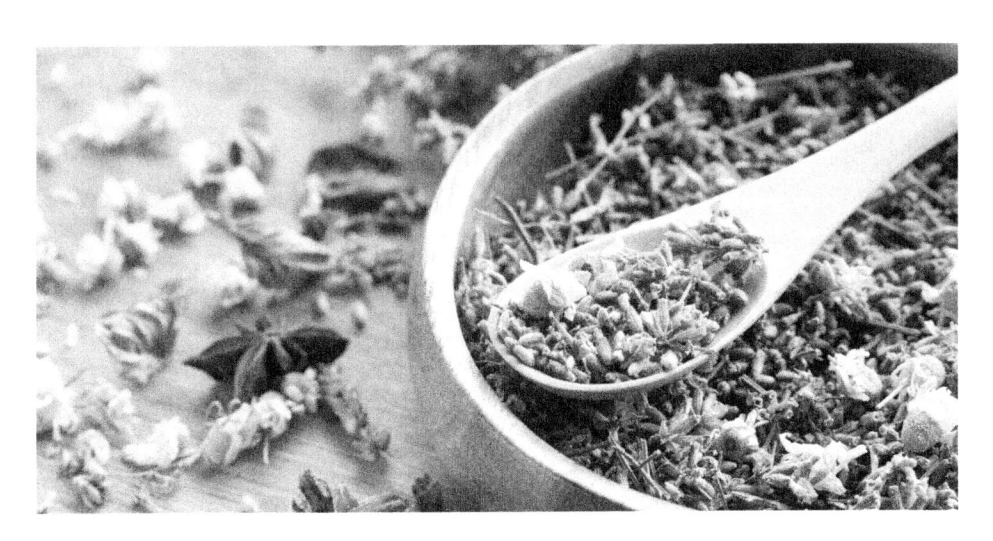

## Chapter 7
# Herbs for the Endocrine/Reproductive System

**Amalaki:** Amalaki is rich in antioxidants that support the health of the endocrine system. It promotes balanced hormone function and aids in the proper functioning of the reproductive organs, helping to maintain overall vitality and hormonal equilibrium.

**Anantmool:** Anantmool is known for balancing hormones and purifying the reproductive system. It helps cleanse and detoxify the reproductive organs while ensuring that hormonal levels remain stable, making it effective for supporting overall reproductive health.

**Ashwagandha:** Ashwagandha is a powerful adaptogenic herb that regulates hormone function and supports adrenal health. It helps manage stress and cortisol levels, which in turn promotes better hormone balance and supports reproductive wellness.

**Bala:** Bala is revered for strengthening reproductive tissues and improving vitality. It nourishes and rejuvenates the reproductive organs, enhancing stamina and ensuring optimal function of the reproductive system, making it particularly beneficial for overall reproductive health.

# Herbs for the Endocrine/Reproductive System

**Fenugreek:** Fenugreek is a versatile herb that helps balance blood sugar levels and supports healthy hormone function. It is especially effective for improving estrogen balance in women and can aid in the management of symptoms associated with hormonal fluctuations.

**Gokshura:** Gokshura is well-known for enhancing reproductive health and boosting vitality. It supports the function of the reproductive organs, improves libido, and helps maintain hormonal balance, making it a popular choice for both men and women.

**Guduchi:** Guduchi strengthens the immune system and supports the endocrine glands. It helps maintain proper hormone levels and supports glandular health, making it essential for a well-functioning endocrine system and reproductive vitality.

**Guggulu:** Guggulu is a key herb for balancing hormones and supporting the thyroid gland. It helps regulate metabolism and ensures that the endocrine system operates smoothly, making it beneficial for overall hormonal health and reproductive function.

**Haritaki:** Haritaki is known for its detoxifying properties that support reproductive organ health. It helps cleanse and purify the reproductive system, promoting better hormonal balance and ensuring optimal function of the endocrine glands.

**Jatamansi:** Jatamansi calms the nervous system and balances the endocrine system. It reduces stress, which helps stabilize hormone production and supports the proper functioning of the reproductive organs, making it a soothing and balancing herb.

# Herbs for the Endocrine/Reproductive System

**Kapikacchu:** Kapikacchu supports reproductive function and balances testosterone levels. It is particularly beneficial for male reproductive health, promoting fertility and enhancing sexual wellness, while also helping to maintain overall hormonal equilibrium.

**Kumari:** Kumari, also known as Aloe Vera, is used to regulate menstrual cycles and support uterine health. It helps balance hormones, reduce menstrual irregularities, and nourish the reproductive organs, promoting overall reproductive wellness.

**Neem:** Neem is known for purifying the blood and regulating hormone function. It supports healthy reproductive and endocrine systems by removing toxins and promoting a balanced hormonal environment, making it effective for reproductive cleansing.

**Punarnava:** Punarnava is helpful in regulating hormones and supporting kidney function. It aids in maintaining hormonal balance, particularly by supporting the adrenal glands, and contributes to overall endocrine and reproductive health.

**Safed Musli:** Safed Musli is a powerful herb that boosts fertility and supports overall reproductive health. It nourishes the reproductive organs, enhances vitality, and balances hormones, making it ideal for improving fertility and sexual wellness.

**Shatavari:** Shatavari is a key herb for balancing hormones and supporting reproductive health in women. It helps regulate estrogen levels, promotes fertility, and nourishes the female reproductive organs, making it essential for women's health.

# Herbs for the Endocrine/Reproductive System

**Triphala:** Triphala is a cleansing blend that supports reproductive and endocrine health. It helps detoxify the body, improve digestive function, and promote a balanced hormonal environment, ensuring optimal reproductive wellness.

**Turmeric:** Turmeric contains curcumin, which is renowned for its anti-inflammatory benefits that support healthy hormone levels. It helps regulate endocrine function, reduce inflammation, and promote overall hormonal balance, benefiting both the reproductive and endocrine systems.

**Vidari Kanda:** Vidari Kanda is known for nourishing the reproductive organs and balancing hormones. It supports sexual health and fertility by strengthening reproductive tissues and promoting hormonal equilibrium, making it a vital herb for reproductive wellness.

**Yashtimadhu:** Yashtimadhu, or Licorice Root, is used to balance hormones and support adrenal function. It helps regulate cortisol levels, soothe the adrenal glands, and promote overall endocrine stability, which in turn supports reproductive health.

## Gear up for a fun-filled challenge and see if you can crack this mind-bending crossword puzzle—let the adventure begin!

Complete the crossword on the next pages or online at AyurvedaPartner.com/HolisticHealingWithHerbs.html.

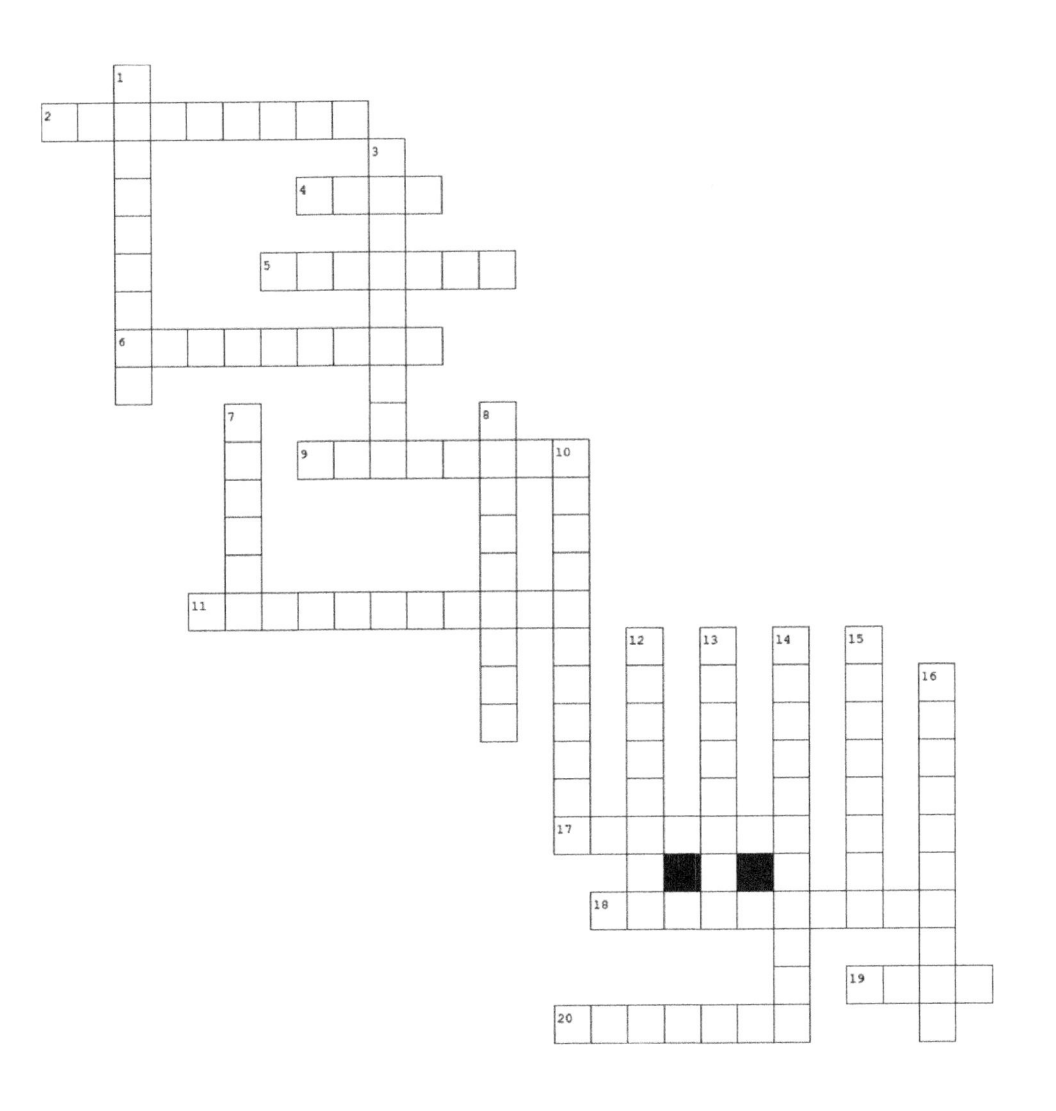

# Herbs for the Endocrine/Reproductive System

# Herbs for the Endocrine/Reproductive System

## Across

2. Balances hormones and purifies the reproductive system
4. Purifies the blood and regulates hormone function
5. Strengthens the immune system and supports the endocrine glands
6. Balances hormones and supports reproductive health in women
9. Enhances reproductive health and boosts vitality
11. Nourishes the reproductive organs and balances hormones (Two words)
17. Provides antioxidants to support endocrine health
18. Supports reproductive function and balances testosterone levels
19. Strengthens reproductive tissues and improves vitality
20. Balances hormones and supports the thyroid gland

## Down

1. Calms the nervous system and balances the endocrine system
3. Balances blood sugar and supports healthy hormone levels
7. Also known as Aloe Vera. Regulates menstrual cycles and supports uterine health
8. Aids in regulating hormones and supports kidney function
10. Regulates hormone function and supports adrenal health
12. Cleanses the body and supports reproductive and endocrine health
13. Detoxifies the body and supports reproductive organ health
14. Balances hormones and supports adrenal function
15. Reduces inflammation and supports healthy hormone levels
16. Boosts fertility and supports overall reproductive health (Two words)

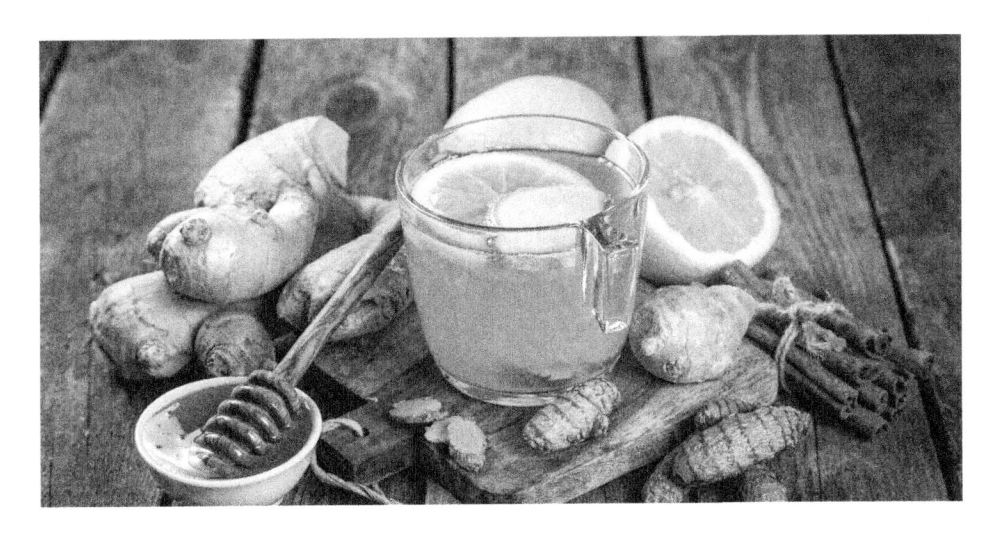

## Chapter 8
# Herbs for the Hematologic/Immunologic System

**Amalaki:** Amalaki is rich in Vitamin C and supports immune health and blood quality. It enhances the production and function of white blood cells, which are crucial for fighting infections, and improves blood circulation, making it a key herb for boosting the immune system.

**Ashwagandha:** Ashwagandha is known for enhancing immune function and supporting healthy white blood cell production. It helps the body adapt to stress, which in turn strengthens immune defenses and promotes overall vitality, protecting against illness.

**Bala:** Bala strengthens the immune system and nourishes the body's tissues. It provides deep nourishment to the blood and supports the body's natural defenses, making it a vital herb for sustaining long-term health and immunity.

**Brahmi:** Brahmi supports the immune system and balances the body's response to stress. By calming the nervous system, it enhances immune resilience and ensures that the body can maintain a robust defense against infections and illnesses.

# Herbs for the Hematologic/Immunologic System

**Guggulu:** Guggulu is known for cleansing the blood and promoting a balanced immune response. It helps detoxify the body and reduces inflammation, supporting the immune system's ability to respond effectively to infections and toxins.

**Guduchi:** Guduchi is a powerful herb that strengthens the immune system and supports overall vitality. It helps cleanse the blood, reduces inflammation, and boosts the body's defenses, making it a key herb for maintaining robust health.

**Haritaki:** Haritaki is a cleansing herb that supports detoxification and enhances immunity. It helps remove toxins from the blood, promoting a healthier immune system and ensuring that the body can effectively combat infections.

**Khadira:** Khadira is renowned for cleansing the blood and supporting skin and immune health. It purifies the bloodstream and reduces inflammatory conditions, making it useful for maintaining a balanced and responsive immune system.

**Kutki:** Kutki is a detoxifying herb that supports liver and immune health. It cleanses the liver, enhances the body's ability to eliminate toxins, and strengthens the immune system, making it effective for protecting the body from infections.

**Licorice Root:** Licorice Root supports immune function and soothes inflammatory conditions. It helps modulate the immune response and reduces inflammation, promoting overall immune resilience and soothing tissues affected by infection or irritation.

# Herbs for the Hematologic/Immunologic System

**Manjistha:** Manjistha purifies the blood and supports the lymphatic system. It helps remove toxins from the bloodstream, boosts immune function, and promotes clear, healthy skin, making it an essential herb for comprehensive detoxification.

**Moringa:** Moringa provides essential nutrients that support immunity and blood health. Rich in vitamins and minerals, it nourishes the blood and strengthens the immune system, ensuring the body has the resources needed to fight off infections.

**Neem:** Neem is a purifying herb that cleanses the blood and supports a healthy immune response. It has strong antibacterial and antiviral properties, making it effective in fighting infections and keeping the immune system balanced.

**Pippali:** Pippali enhances immune function and purifies the respiratory tract. It stimulates immune defenses and helps clear mucus from the lungs, making it a valuable herb for respiratory and overall immune health.

**Punarnava:** Punarnava is a rejuvenating herb that purifies the blood and supports healthy kidney function. It helps remove excess fluid and toxins from the body, enhancing immune efficiency and supporting overall vitality.

**Shatavari:** Shatavari nourishes the blood and enhances immune function. It helps balance hormones and strengthen the body's defenses, making it a valuable herb for women's health and overall immune support.

# Herbs for the Hematologic/Immunologic System

**Trikatu:** Trikatu is a combination that enhances immune function and promotes detoxification. It helps stimulate digestion and clear toxins from the body, ensuring the immune system remains strong and responsive.

**Triphala:** Triphala detoxifies the blood and supports a healthy immune system. It cleanses the digestive tract and promotes the elimination of waste, strengthening immune function and maintaining overall health.

**Tulsi:** Tulsi, also known as Holy Basil, boosts immunity and helps purify the blood. It has powerful antiviral and antibacterial properties, making it effective in protecting against infections and promoting respiratory health.

**Turmeric:** Turmeric contains curcumin, which has powerful anti-inflammatory and immune-boosting properties. It supports the body's natural defenses and helps keep the immune system balanced, making it an essential herb for maintaining health and preventing disease.

## Put your brainpower to the test and see if you can master this intriguing crossword puzzle—how many clues can you conquer?

Complete the crossword on the next pages or online at AyurvedaPartner.com/HolisticHealingWithHerbs.html.

# Herbs for the Hematologic/Immunologic System

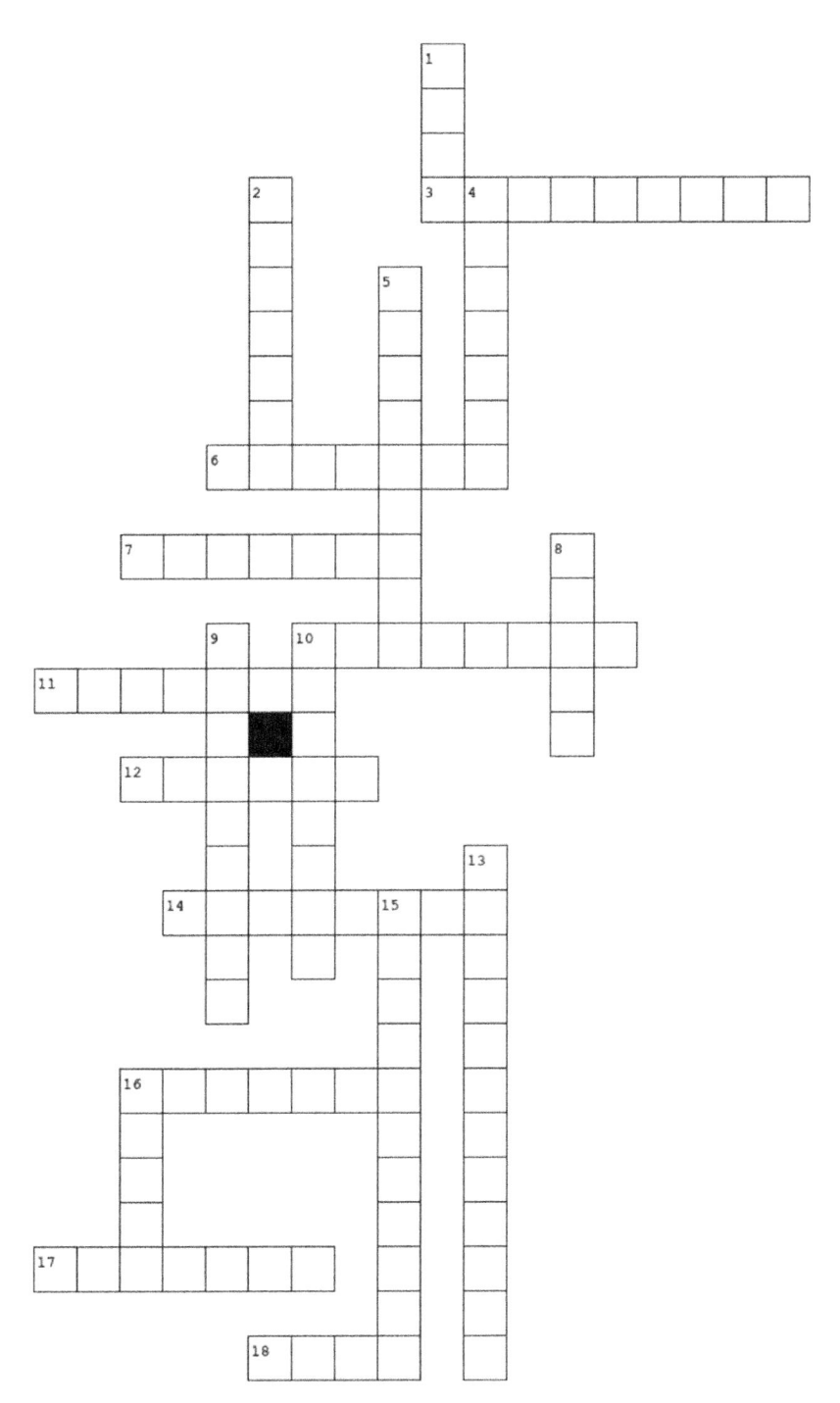

# Herbs for the Hematologic/Immunologic System

**Across**

3. Purifies the blood and supports the lymphatic system
6. Enhances immune function and purifies the respiratory tract
7. Provides essential nutrients that support immunity and blood health
10. Detoxifies the blood and supports a healthy immune system
11. Cleanses the blood and promotes a balanced immune response
12. Supports the immune system and balances the body's response to stress
14. Supports detoxification and enhances immunity
16. Cleanses the blood and supports skin and immune health
17. A combination that enhances immune function and promotes detoxification
18. Strengthens the immune system and nourishes the body's tissues

**Down**

1. Purifies the blood and supports a healthy immune response
2. Strengthens the immune system and supports overall vitality
4. Rich in Vitamin C and supports immune health and blood quality
5. Nourishes the blood and enhances immune function
8. Boosts immunity and helps purify the blood
9. Purifies the blood and supports healthy kidney function
10. Contains curcumin, which has powerful anti-inflammatory and immune-boosting properties
13. Supports immune function and soothes inflammatory conditions (Two words)
15. Enhances immune function and supports healthy white blood cell production
16. Detoxifies the liver and supports immune health

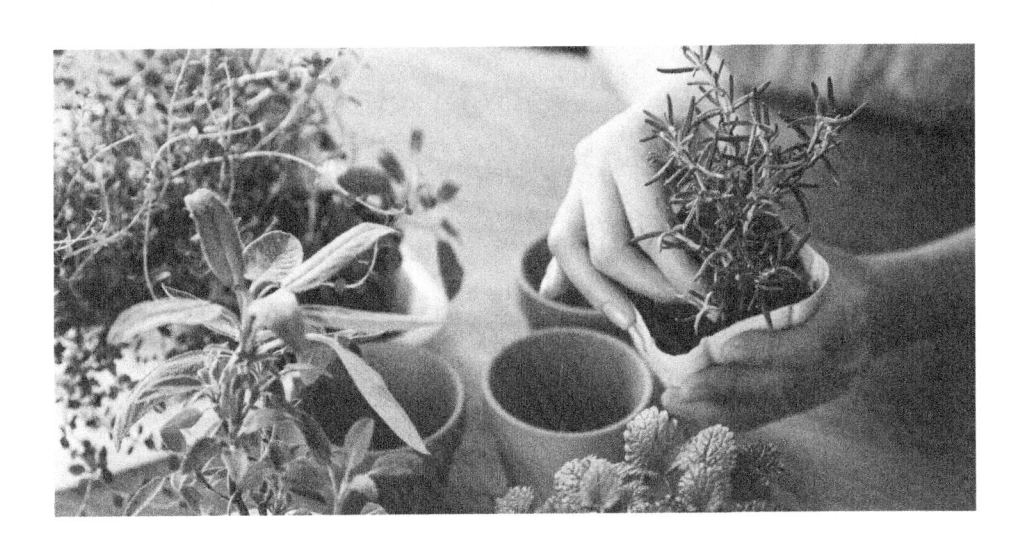

## Chapter 9
# Herbs for the Skin

**Amalaki:** Amalaki is packed with Vitamin C, which supports collagen production and enhances skin vitality. It helps rejuvenate the skin from within, reducing fine lines and promoting a youthful, glowing complexion.

**Ashwagandha:** Ashwagandha is known for reducing stress-related skin issues and improving elasticity. It combats the effects of stress on the skin, helping to maintain a firm and smooth appearance while reducing the signs of aging.

**Bala:** Bala is a nourishing herb that rejuvenates the skin tissues. It enhances the skin's natural glow and promotes healthy hydration, making the skin feel supple and resilient to environmental stressors.

**Brahmi:** Brahmi has calming properties that soothe the skin and reduce irritation and inflammation. It nourishes the skin, helping to relieve conditions such as redness, eczema, and rashes, promoting an even and calm complexion.

# Herbs for the Skin

**Calendula:** Calendula is widely recognized for its ability to heal and soothe irritated skin. It reduces inflammation, promotes rapid wound healing, and leaves the skin feeling soft and comfortable, making it ideal for sensitive or damaged skin.

**Castor Oil:** Castor Oil hydrates the skin and supports healing of dry, cracked areas. Its deeply moisturizing properties help soothe rough patches and repair skin damage, leaving the skin feeling nourished and smooth.

**Gotu Kola:** Gotu Kola improves skin tone and promotes wound healing. It stimulates collagen synthesis, which enhances skin firmness and reduces the appearance of scars and blemishes, giving the skin a more even and healthy look.

**Guduchi:** Guduchi is a rejuvenating herb that supports skin health and reduces irritation. It helps purify the skin, soothe redness, and prevent breakouts, leaving the skin looking refreshed and healthy.

**Khadira:** Khadira is effective for clearing skin issues like eczema and psoriasis. It has purifying and astringent properties that soothe inflammatory skin conditions and promote a clear and balanced complexion.

**Kumari:** Kumari, also known as Aloe Vera, hydrates and rejuvenates the skin from within. It helps retain moisture, soothes irritation, and leaves the skin feeling refreshed and supple, making it a must-have for daily skincare.

# Herbs for the Skin

**Manjistha:** Manjistha detoxifies the blood and promotes glowing skin. It works from the inside out to reduce blemishes, clear up acne, and leave the skin with a naturally radiant and even complexion.

**Neem:** Neem is a purifying herb that cleanses the blood and promotes clear, healthy skin. It helps combat acne, reduces excess oil, and prevents infections, making it a powerful remedy for achieving smooth and blemish-free skin.

**Nirgundi:** Nirgundi reduces skin inflammation and soothes irritation. It is particularly beneficial for relieving itchy and inflamed skin conditions, providing a calming effect that restores the skin's natural balance.

**Saffron:** Saffron is prized for improving complexion and reducing blemishes. It brightens the skin, evens out skin tone, and helps diminish the appearance of dark spots, giving the skin a luminous and flawless look.

**Sandalwood:** Sandalwood is known for its calming properties, which soothe skin irritation and improve complexion. It reduces redness and cools the skin, leaving it feeling smooth and refreshed, with a soft, natural glow.

**Triphala:** Triphala detoxifies the skin and promotes a natural glow. It helps cleanse the body from within, clearing toxins that can cause breakouts, and leaves the skin looking vibrant and revitalized.

# Herbs for the Skin

**Tulsi:** Tulsi is a potent herb for fighting skin infections and purifying the skin. It has antibacterial and antifungal properties that keep the skin clear, reduce blemishes, and enhance the skin's overall radiance.

**Turmeric:** Turmeric is renowned for reducing inflammation and enhancing skin radiance. It brightens the skin, evens out skin tone, and reduces redness, making it a powerful remedy for achieving a healthy, glowing complexion.

**Vetiver:** Vetiver is a cooling herb that soothes inflamed skin and reduces redness. It hydrates and nourishes the skin, leaving it feeling calm, refreshed, and balanced, making it perfect for sensitive or overheated skin.

**Yashtimadhu:** Yashtimadhu, also known as Licorice Root, brightens the skin and soothes redness and irritation. It helps reduce dark spots and hyperpigmentation, promoting a clearer and more even complexion.

## Unlock your inner puzzle master and embark on this exciting crossword challenge—can you solve every clue and complete the grid?

Complete the crossword on the next pages or online at AyurvedaPartner.com/HolisticHealingWithHerbs.html.

# Herbs for the Skin

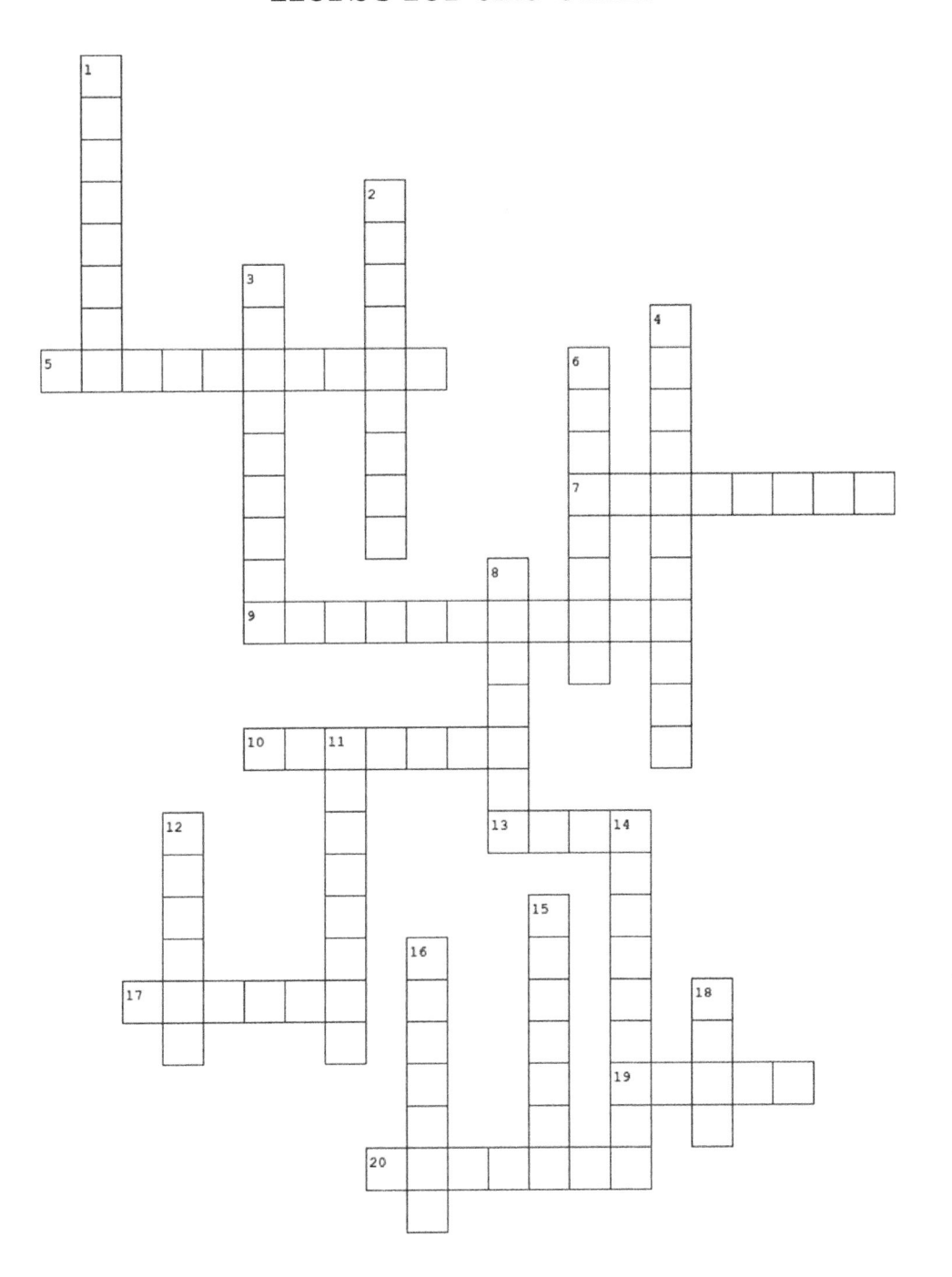

# Herbs for the Skin

## Across

5. Calms skin irritation and improves skin complexion

7. Improves skin tone and promotes wound healing (Two words)

9. Reduces stress-related skin issues and improves elasticity

10. Cools and soothes inflamed skin, reducing redness

13. Purifies the blood and promotes clear, healthy skin

17. Calms the skin and reduces irritation and inflammation

19. Fights skin infections and purifies the skin

20. Clears skin issues like eczema and psoriasis

## Down

1. Detoxifies the skin and promotes a natural glow

2. Hydrates the skin and supports healing of dry, cracked areas (Two words)

3. Heals and soothes irritated skin

4. Brightens skin and soothes redness and irritation

6. Reduces skin inflammation and soothes irritation

8. Improves complexion and reduces blemishes

11. Reduces inflammation and enhances skin radiance

12. Hydrates and rejuvenates the skin from within

14. Detoxifies the blood and promotes glowing skin

15. Rich in Vitamin C, supports collagen production and skin vitality

16. Supports skin health and reduces skin irritation

18. Nourishes and rejuvenates the skin tissues

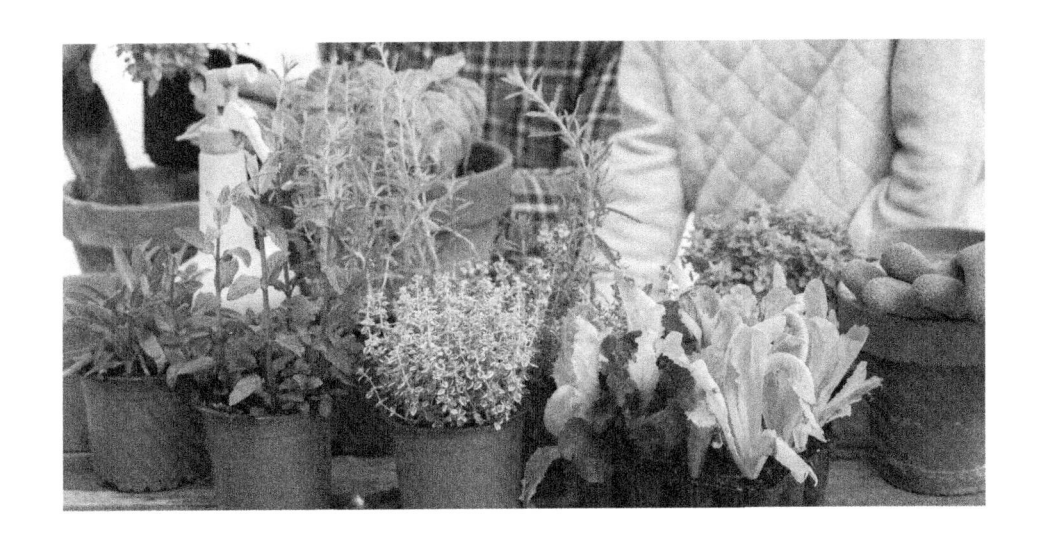

## Chapter 10
# Herbs for the Nervous System

**Anantmool:** Anantmool is a calming herb that soothes the nervous system and supports mental health. It helps alleviate stress and anxiety, promoting emotional balance and a sense of overall well-being, making it essential for maintaining a peaceful mind.

**Gotu Kola:** Gotu Kola is a powerful herb that supports brain health and enhances cognitive function. It boosts memory, improves concentration, and strengthens the nervous system, making it an ideal tonic for mental clarity and focus.

**Guggulu:** Guggulu is known for protecting the nerves and reducing oxidative stress. It helps maintain the integrity of the nervous system by combating free radical damage, promoting healthy nerve function, and reducing inflammation.

# Herbs for the Nervous System

**Jyotishmati:** Jyotishmati is revered for promoting mental clarity and strengthening the nervous system. It sharpens memory, enhances concentration, and supports a balanced mind, making it a key herb for mental and cognitive wellness.

**Kali Musli:** Kali Musli is an herb that strengthens the nerves and promotes mental stability. It helps reduce anxiety and nervous tension, providing a sense of calm and balance while supporting the overall resilience of the nervous system.

**Kava Kava:** Kava Kava is well-known for promoting relaxation and calming the nervous system. It helps relieve stress and anxiety, providing a tranquilizing effect that encourages a sense of peace and emotional well-being.

**Licorice Root:** Licorice Root balances the nervous system and soothes inflammation. It supports adrenal health, reduces stress, and promotes a relaxed state, making it useful for calming an overactive nervous system.

**Mandukaparni:** Mandukaparni enhances brain function and balances mental activity. It promotes mental sharpness, reduces stress, and supports healthy circulation to the brain, making it valuable for cognitive health and emotional stability.

**Mucuna Pruriens:** Mucuna Pruriens is known for boosting dopamine levels and supporting nervous system health. It helps improve mood, reduce stress, and enhance mental alertness, making it a beneficial herb for emotional and neurological well-being.

# Herbs for the Nervous System

**Nutmeg:** Nutmeg is a calming herb that soothes the mind and promotes deep, restful sleep. It reduces nervous tension and anxiety, making it ideal for relaxation and rejuvenation of the nervous system.

**Pippali:** Pippali improves brain function and supports nervous clarity. It enhances the flow of oxygen to the brain, sharpens cognitive abilities, and calms the mind, contributing to overall nervous system health.

**Shatavari:** Shatavari nourishes the nervous system and balances emotions. It provides a grounding effect, helps manage stress, and supports emotional stability, making it a key herb for soothing and rejuvenating the mind.

**Tagara:** Tagara is known for relaxing the nervous system and promoting restful sleep. It helps ease anxiety and nervousness, making it a natural remedy for insomnia and supporting a calm and balanced state of mind.

**Tulsi:** Tulsi is an adaptogenic herb that reduces nervous tension and supports mental focus. It calms the mind, enhances concentration, and provides resilience against stress, promoting a balanced and healthy nervous system.

# Herbs for the Nervous System

**Turmeric:** Turmeric is celebrated for reducing neuroinflammation and supporting brain health. It helps protect the nervous system from degenerative diseases and promotes cognitive function, making it essential for maintaining a healthy brain.

**Vacha:** Vacha calms the mind and supports speech and nervous clarity. It helps clear mental fog, enhances verbal expression, and soothes the nervous system, making it valuable for clear communication and a calm mind.

## Dive into the fun and test your skills with this captivating crossword puzzle —can you solve it all?

Complete the crossword on the next pages or online at AyurvedaPartner.com/HolisticHealingWithHerbs.html.

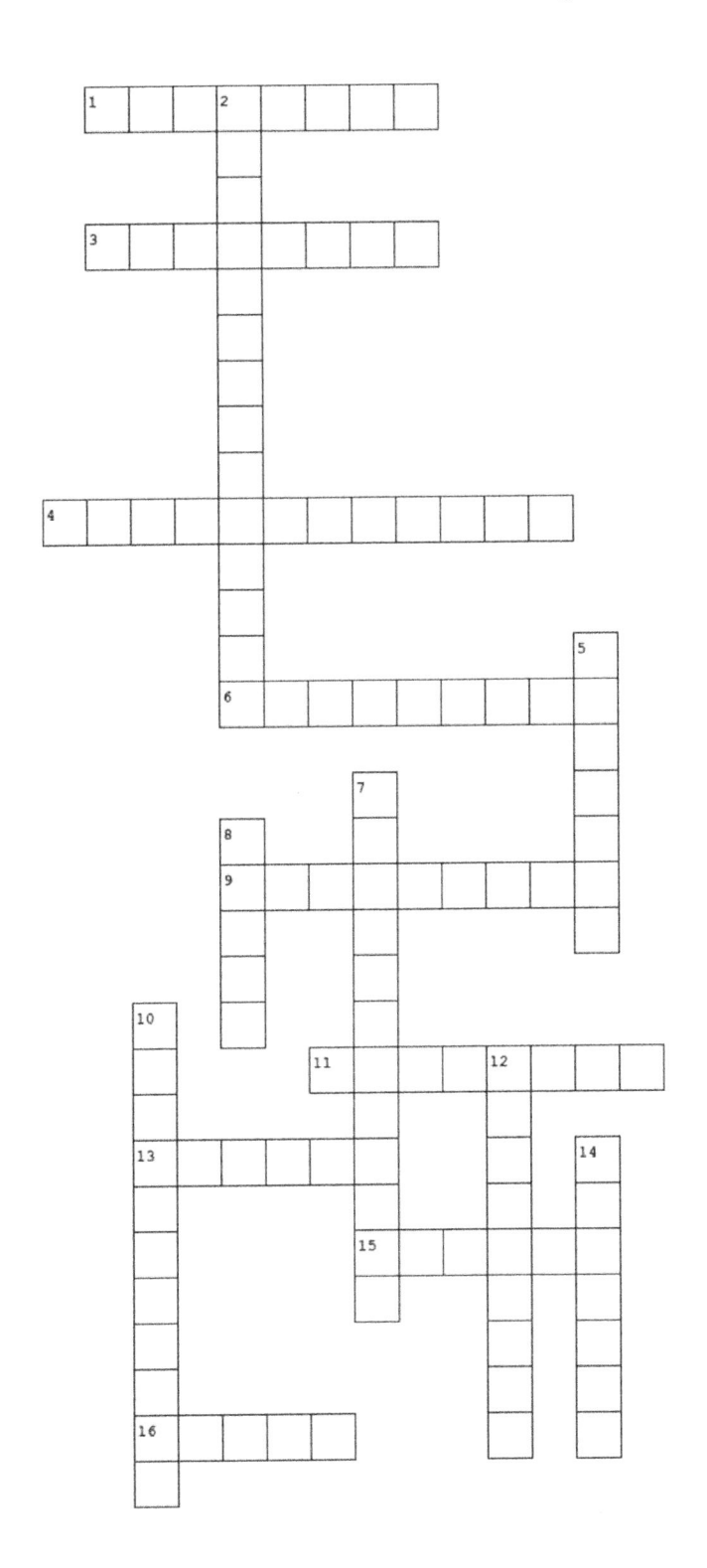

# Herbs for the Nervous System

# Herbs for the Nervous System

**Across**

1. Reduces neuroinflammation and supports brain health
3. Supports brain health and enhances cognitive function (Two words)
4. Balances the nervous system and soothes inflammation (Two words)
6. Nourishes the nervous system and balances emotions
9. Calms the nervous system and supports mental health
11. Promotes relaxation and calms the nervous system (Two words)
13. Relaxes the nervous system and promotes restful sleep
15. Calms the mind and promotes deep, restful sleep
16. Reduces nervous tension and supports mental focus

**Down**

2. Boosts dopamine levels and supports nervous system health (Two words)
5. Improves brain function and supports nervous clarity
7. Enhances brain function and balances mental activity
8. Calms the mind and supports speech and nervous clarity
10. Promotes mental clarity and strengthens the nervous system
12. Strengthens the nerves and promotes mental stability (Two words)
14. Protects the nerves and reduces oxidative stress

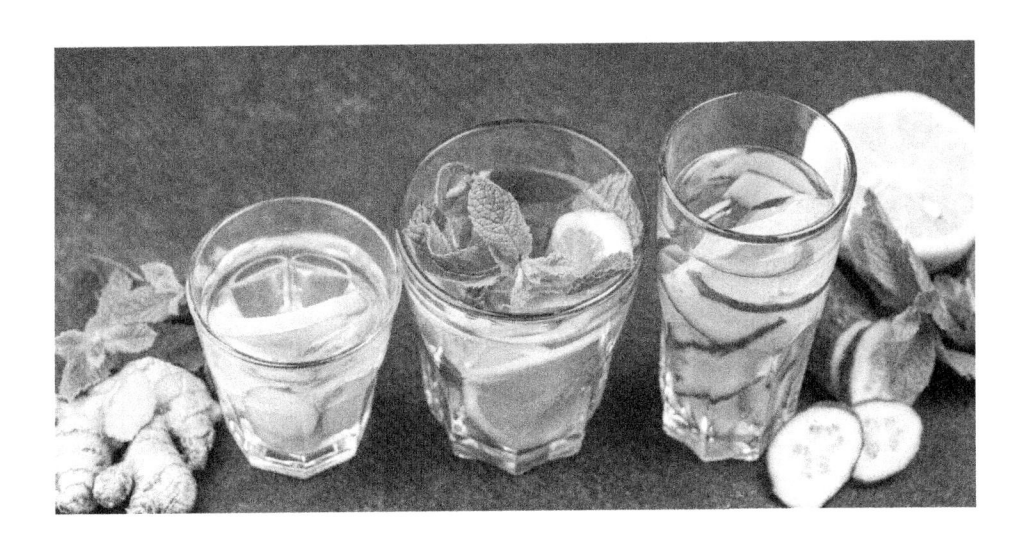

## Chapter 11
# Herbs that Detoxify

**Aloe Vera:** Aloe Vera is known for cleansing the digestive tract and supporting bowel movements. It acts as a natural laxative, gently flushing out toxins and promoting regularity, which helps maintain a healthy and detoxified digestive system.

**Amalaki:** Amalaki is rich in antioxidants that cleanse the body and support digestion. It aids in the removal of free radicals and waste from the body, helping to rejuvenate the digestive system and promote overall detoxification.

**Ashwagandha:** Ashwagandha detoxifies the tissues and supports adrenal health. It helps eliminate toxins from the deeper tissues, rejuvenates the body, and balances stress hormones, ensuring that the body's detoxification processes remain efficient.

**Basil:** Basil supports respiratory detoxification and purifies the blood. It helps clear mucus from the lungs, eliminates impurities from the bloodstream, and provides a cleansing effect on the respiratory system, aiding overall detoxification.

# Herbs that Detoxify

**Bhumyamalaki:** Bhumyamalaki protects the liver and aids in removing toxins. It supports liver function, helps cleanse the bloodstream, and promotes the elimination of harmful substances, making it a powerful detoxifying herb.

**Burdock Root:** Burdock Root purifies the blood and supports liver function. It helps remove toxins through the skin and kidneys, clears impurities from the bloodstream, and promotes a healthy and cleansed internal environment.

**Chitrak:** Chitrak supports metabolic fire and aids in clearing toxins from the digestive tract. It helps ignite the digestive system, break down waste, and eliminate toxins, ensuring that the body's metabolism remains strong and efficient.

**Cilantro:** Cilantro is well-known for helping to remove heavy metals from the body and supporting digestion. It binds to toxic metals and assists in their elimination, while also promoting a healthy digestive system to support detoxification.

**Coriander:** Coriander removes heavy metals and balances the digestive fire. It supports the natural cleansing processes of the liver and kidneys, helping the body efficiently expel toxins while promoting digestive balance.

**Fennel:** Fennel aids in digestion and helps flush out toxins from the system. It soothes the digestive tract, reduces bloating, and enhances the elimination of waste, making it an effective herb for gentle detoxification.

# Herbs that Detoxify

**Guggulu:** Guggulu purifies the blood and promotes the elimination of metabolic waste. It helps break down toxins and excess fat, aiding in the body's natural cleansing processes and supporting overall metabolic health.

**Guduchi:** Guduchi enhances liver function and helps eliminate toxins. It supports the immune system, reduces inflammation, and promotes the removal of waste products from the liver and other vital organs, aiding in overall detoxification.

**Haritaki:** Haritaki gently purges toxins from the colon and supports digestion. It cleanses the gastrointestinal tract, promotes regular bowel movements, and helps remove waste and toxins from the digestive system, ensuring a clean and healthy gut.

**Kutki:** Kutki supports liver and gallbladder function and aids in detoxification. It helps cleanse the liver, promotes bile flow, and enhances the elimination of toxins, making it effective for detoxifying the body's primary filtration systems.

**Manjistha:** Manjistha detoxifies the lymphatic system and promotes healthy blood flow. It clears impurities from the lymphatic system, purifies the blood, and supports healthy circulation, ensuring the body's waste removal processes are functioning well.

**Neem:** Neem purifies the blood and supports liver and kidney detoxification. It helps eliminate toxins from the bloodstream, supports liver health, and promotes the body's ability to cleanse itself naturally, keeping the immune system strong.

# Herbs that Detoxify

**Pippali:** Pippali enhances lung detoxification and boosts metabolism. It helps clear respiratory toxins, supports digestion, and promotes healthy metabolic processes, making it an excellent herb for full-body detoxification.

**Punarnava:** Punarnava is known for cleansing the kidneys and reducing water retention. It helps eliminate excess fluids and toxins from the body, supports kidney health, and promotes a healthy urinary system, aiding in overall detoxification.

**Triphala:** Triphala, a blend of three fruits, cleanses the digestive system and detoxifies the body. It promotes regular bowel movements, removes toxins from the intestines, and rejuvenates the gut, making it a foundational Ayurvedic remedy for detoxification.

**Turmeric:** Turmeric contains curcumin, which supports liver detoxification and reduces inflammation. It helps the liver process and eliminate toxins while also promoting a healthy inflammatory response, making it an essential herb for detoxification and overall well-being.

## Prepare to ignite your mind and tackle this thrilling crossword adventure—can you master it?

Complete the crossword on the next pages or online at AyurvedaPartner.com/HolisticHealingWithHerbs.html.

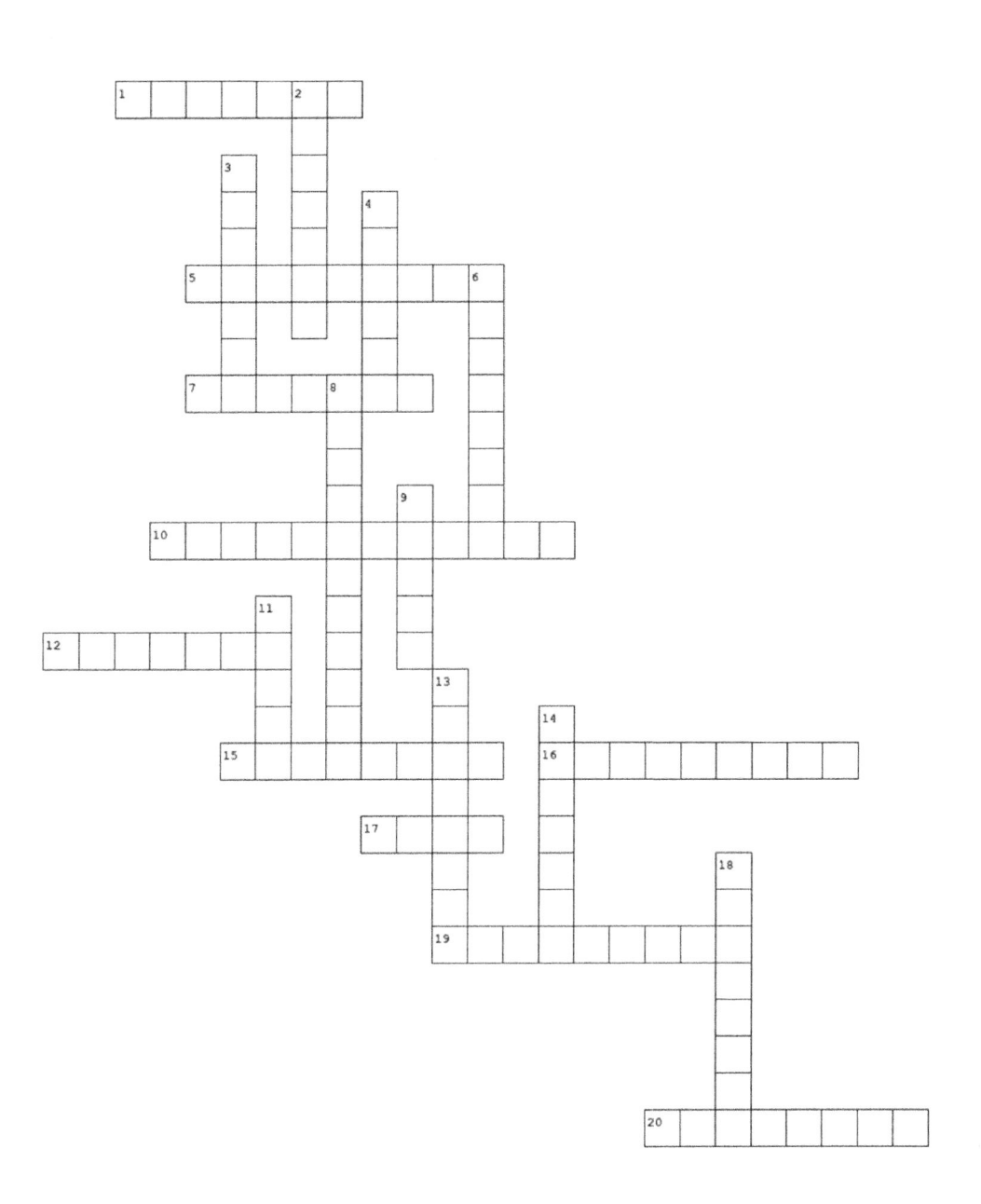

# Herbs that Detoxify

# Herbs that Detoxify

**Across**

1. Root Purifies the blood and supports liver function
5. Cleanses the kidneys and reduces water retention
7. Enhances lung detoxification and boosts metabolism
10. Protects the liver and aids in removing toxins
12. Purifies the blood and promotes the elimination of metabolic waste
15. Helps remove heavy metals from the body and supports digestion
16. Detoxifies the lymphatic system and promotes healthy blood flow
17. Purifies the blood and supports liver and kidney detoxification
19. Removes heavy metals and balances the digestive fire
20. A blend of three fruits that cleanses the digestive system and detoxifies the body

**Down**

2. Supports metabolic fire and aids in clearing toxins from the digestive tract
3. Enhances liver function and helps eliminate toxins
4. Aids in digestion and helps flush out toxins from the system
6. Cleanses the digestive tract and supports bowel movements (Two words)
8. Detoxifies the tissues and supports adrenal health
9. Supports respiratory detoxification and purifies the blood
11. Supports liver and gallbladder function and aids in detoxification
13. Supports liver detoxification and reduces inflammation
14. Rich in antioxidants that cleanse the body and support digestion
18. Gently purges toxins from the colon and supports digestion

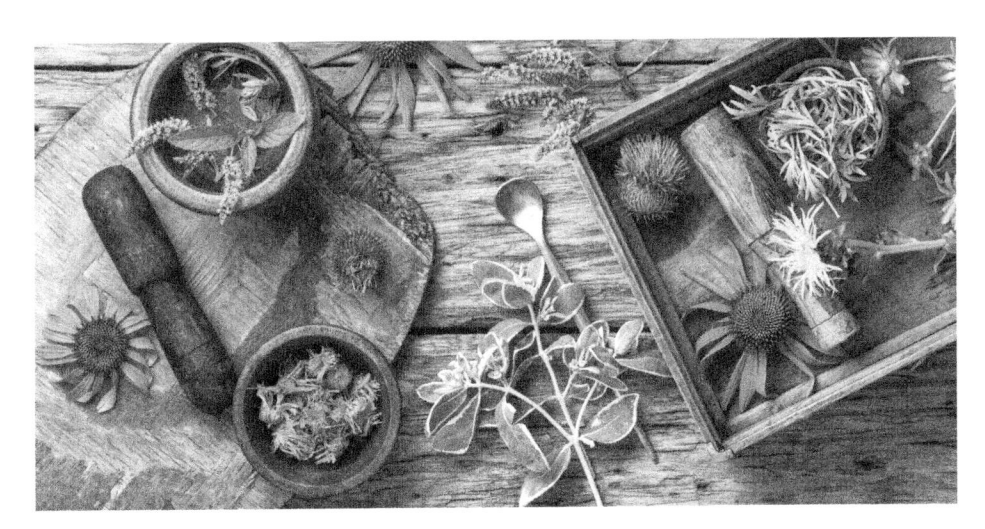

## Chapter 12
# Herbs for Emotional/Mental Well-being

**Ashwagandha:** Adaptogen known to reduce stress and anxiety, Ashwagandha helps regulate cortisol levels, enhancing emotional resilience and promoting a sense of calm. It is valued for boosting mental clarity, focus, and overall well-being, making it an ideal choice for combating chronic stress and burnout.

**Brahmi:** Enhances memory and cognitive function while calming the nervous system. Brahmi is widely used to alleviate anxiety, sharpen intellect, and foster a sense of inner peace. It reduces oxidative stress in the brain, supporting long-term cognitive health and emotional stability.

**Gotu Kola:** Improves concentration and calms the mind. Gotu Kola is renowned for enhancing mental clarity, easing anxiety, and promoting a sense of mindfulness. It is particularly effective for reducing mental fatigue and fostering inner stillness, making it useful for meditation and focus.

# Herbs for Emotional/Mental Well-being

**Holy Basil:** Sacred herb used to uplift mood and combat stress. Holy Basil, or Tulsi, balances hormones and provides relief from emotional and physical exhaustion. It is known for its calming and grounding effects, fostering emotional resilience, improving clarity, and reducing anxiety.

**Shankhpushpi:** Traditional tonic for anxiety and mental fatigue, Shankhpushpi is praised for its ability to soothe an overactive mind and promote restful sleep. It enhances cognitive function, alleviates anxiety, and supports emotional stability, making it a valuable tool for mental harmony.

**Jatamansi:** Herb used for calming the nervous system. Jatamansi is known for reducing anxiety, balancing emotional disturbances, and supporting healthy sleep patterns. It helps manage irritability and anger, fostering a sense of emotional equilibrium and relaxation.

**Valerian:** Known for promoting relaxation and sleep, Valerian is effective in calming the central nervous system and easing muscle tension. It alleviates feelings of restlessness and nervous excitement, making it ideal for those with anxiety-related sleep disturbances.

**Chamomile:** Soothing herb often used in calming teas, Chamomile is well-known for reducing stress and anxiety. Its gentle sedative properties promote restful sleep, ease digestive discomfort caused by stress, and help maintain emotional balance and relaxation.

**Lavender:** Aromatic flower that alleviates stress and anxiety. Lavender is used to calm the nervous system, reduce cortisol levels, and promote relaxation. Its soothing aroma is popular in aromatherapy to uplift the mood and encourage emotional well-being.

# Herbs for Emotional/Mental Well-being

**Lemon Balm:** Uplifts mood and eases tension. Lemon Balm is a gentle herb that calms an overactive mind, reduces irritability, and improves focus. It is often used to relieve anxiety and sleeplessness, creating a sense of inner peace and well-being.

**Rhodiola:** Adaptogen that boosts energy and reduces fatigue. Rhodiola enhances the body's resilience to stress, supports brain function, and balances serotonin and dopamine levels. It is beneficial for combating mental and emotional exhaustion while improving mood and focus.

**Ginkgo Biloba:** Improves blood flow to the brain and memory. Ginkgo Biloba enhances cognitive performance, reduces anxiety, and protects against oxidative damage. It supports emotional stability and mental sharpness, making it useful for boosting focus and clarity.

**Passionflower:** Known for its calming effects on anxiety, Passionflower promotes relaxation by increasing GABA production in the brain. It helps ease nervous tension, soothe a racing mind, and improve sleep, fostering a sense of inner calm and well-being.

**Skullcap:** Helps soothe a racing mind and promotes relaxation. Skullcap calms the nervous system and alleviates chronic stress, reducing emotional overwhelm and promoting restful sleep. It is a valuable herb for achieving mental and emotional balance.

**Rosemary:** Stimulates cognitive function and memory. Rosemary is known for its invigorating effects, enhancing mental clarity, reducing fatigue, and lifting the spirits. Its aromatic properties also promote a positive mood and support emotional well-being.

# Herbs for Emotional/Mental Well-being

**Kava Kava:** Plant used to ease anxiety and promote calm. Kava Kava has potent relaxing properties that reduce symptoms of anxiety and encourage a tranquil state. It is especially effective for social anxiety, fostering a sense of comfort and emotional balance.

**Hops:** Herb known for its sedative and calming properties. Hops is used to promote restful sleep and ease anxiety. It calms the nervous system and reduces restlessness, making it particularly effective for stress-induced tension and deep relaxation.

**Peppermint:** Invigorates the senses and reduces mental fatigue. Peppermint provides a refreshing and energizing effect, alleviating headaches and soothing tension. It enhances focus, clears mental fog, and refreshes the mind for improved clarity.

**Saffron:** Precious spice known to uplift mood and spirit. Saffron contains active compounds that boost serotonin levels, reducing symptoms of depression and anxiety. It promotes a positive outlook, emotional balance, and a sense of happiness.

**Lemon Verbena:** Herb known for its calming and uplifting properties. Lemon Verbena helps reduce anxiety, soothe nervous tension, and promote relaxation. Its citrusy aroma uplifts the spirit, eases mental fatigue, and supports mental clarity and emotional well-being.

# Herbs for Emotional/Mental Well-being

**Rhodiola:** Rhodiola is an adaptogen that boosts energy and reduces fatigue, making it an excellent herb for combating mental and emotional exhaustion. It enhances the body's resilience to stress and supports optimal brain function, improving focus and mood. Rhodiola is also known to balance serotonin and dopamine levels, fostering a positive outlook and emotional stability. It is particularly beneficial for those dealing with stress-induced fatigue.

**Ginkgo Biloba:** Ginkgo Biloba improves blood flow to the brain and memory, enhancing cognitive performance and reducing symptoms of anxiety and depression. It helps protect the brain from oxidative damage and improves concentration and mental clarity. By supporting healthy brain function, Ginkgo Biloba fosters emotional balance and reduces the impact of stress on the nervous system. It is often used to boost focus and mental sharpness.

**Passionflower:** Passionflower is known for its calming effects on anxiety, providing natural relief from restlessness and an overactive mind. It enhances GABA production in the brain, promoting relaxation and easing nervous tension. Passionflower is particularly beneficial for those who experience racing thoughts or have difficulty sleeping due to anxiety. It fosters a sense of inner calm and helps soothe the mind.

**Skullcap:** Skullcap helps soothe a racing mind and promotes relaxation, offering support for those who experience chronic stress or anxiety. This herb is known for its grounding effects, calming the nervous system and reducing emotional overwhelm. Skullcap is particularly useful for managing nervous tension and promoting restful sleep, making it a valuable ally for emotional and mental well-being.

# Herbs for Emotional/Mental Well-being

**Pippali:** Pippali enhances lung detoxification and boosts metabolism. It helps clear respiratory toxins, supports digestion, and promotes healthy metabolic processes, making it an excellent herb for full-body detoxification.

**Punarnava:** Punarnava is known for cleansing the kidneys and reducing water retention. It helps eliminate excess fluids and toxins from the body, supports kidney health, and promotes a healthy urinary system, aiding in overall detoxification.

**Triphala:** Triphala, a blend of three fruits, cleanses the digestive system and detoxifies the body. It promotes regular bowel movements, removes toxins from the intestines, and rejuvenates the gut, making it a foundational Ayurvedic remedy for detoxification.

**Turmeric:** Turmeric contains curcumin, which supports liver detoxification and reduces inflammation. It helps the liver process and eliminate toxins while also promoting a healthy inflammatory response, making it an essential herb for detoxification and overall well-being.

## Challenge your wits and dive into this captivating crossword—will you emerge victorious?

Complete the crossword on the next pages or online at AyurvedaPartner.com/HolisticHealingWithHerbs.html.

# Herbs for Emotional/Mental Well-being

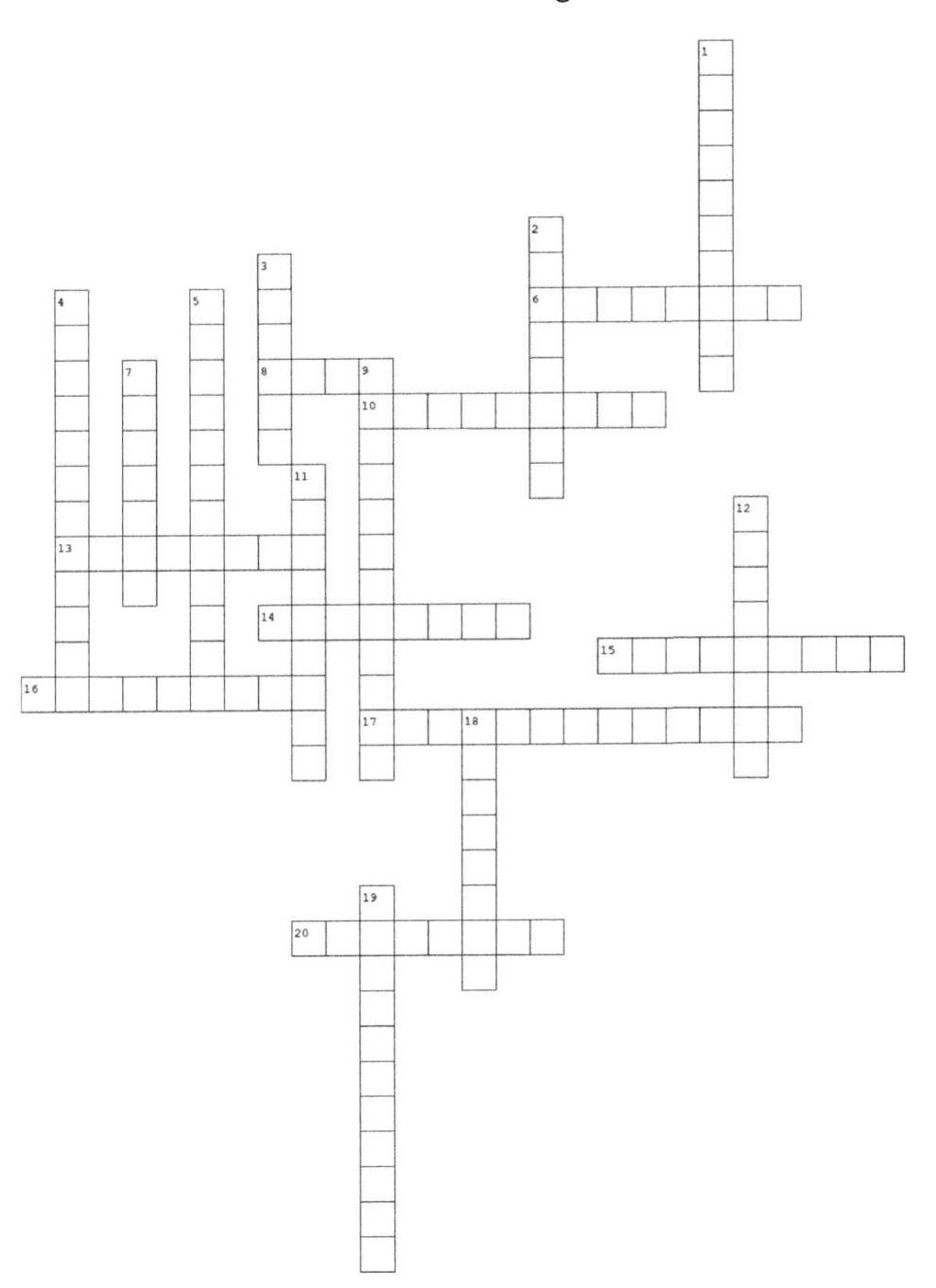

# Herbs for Emotional/Mental Well-being

## Across

6. Known for promoting relaxation and sleep
8. Herb known for its sedative and calming properties
10. Sacred herb used to uplift mood and combat stress (Two words)
13. Adaptogen that boosts energy and reduces fatigue
14. Improves concentration and calms the mind (Two words)
15. Uplifts mood and eases tension (Two words)
16. Herb used for calming the nervous system
17. Known for its calming effects on anxiety
20. Stimulates cognitive function and memory

## Down

1. Invigorates the senses and reduces mental fatigue
2. Plant used to ease anxiety and promote calm (Two words)
3. Enhances memory and cognitive function
4. Herb known for its calming and uplifting properties (Two words)
5. Improves blood flow to the brain and memory (Two words)
7. Precious spice known to uplift mood and spirit
9. Traditional tonic for anxiety and mental fatigue
11. Soothing herb often used in calming teas
12. Aromatic flower that alleviates stress and anxiety
18. Helps soothe a racing mind and promotes relaxation
19. Adaptogen known to reduce stress and anxiety

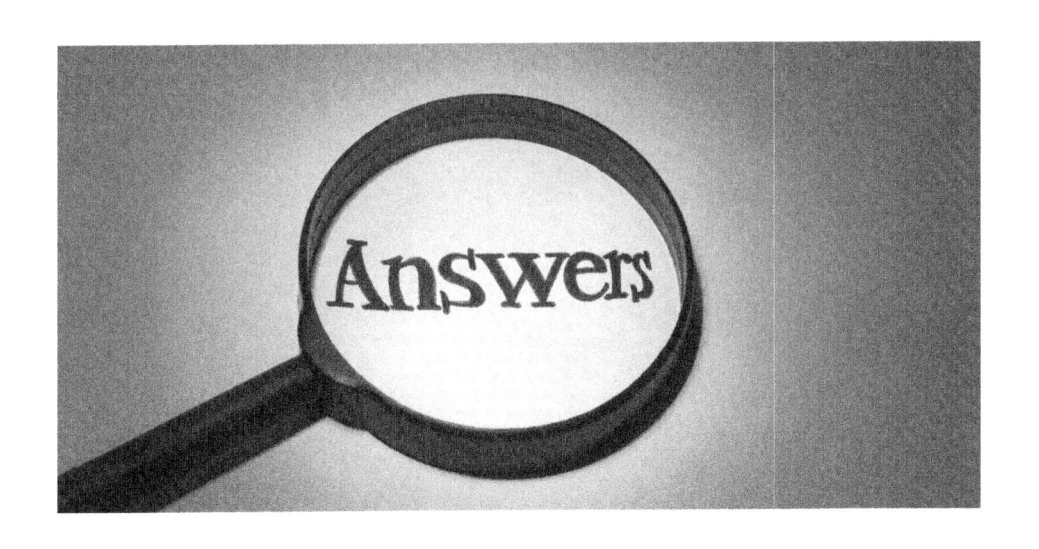

Crossword Puzzle Answer Keys

# Chapter 1
# Common Single Herbs Answer Key

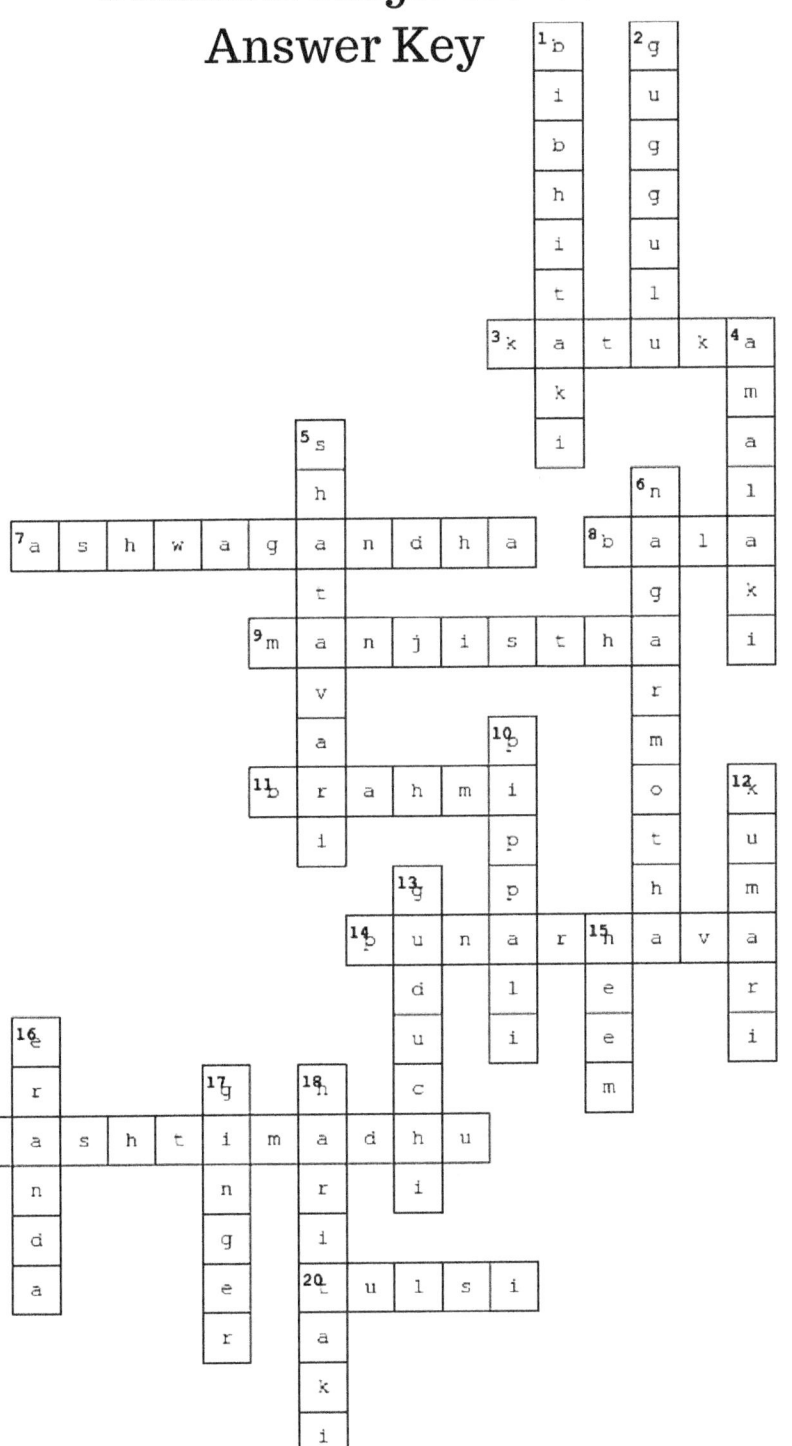

**Across:**
3. katuki
7. ashwagandha
8. bala
9. manjistha
11. brahmi
14. punarhava (punar + hava)
19. yashtimadhu
20. tulsi

**Down:**
1. bibhitaki
2. guggulu
4. amalaki
5. shatavati
6. neem
10. pippali
12. kumari
13. ginger
15. hemeel
16. eranda
17. ginger
18. haridri

81

## Chapter 2
# Herbs for the Gastrointestinal System
## Answer Key

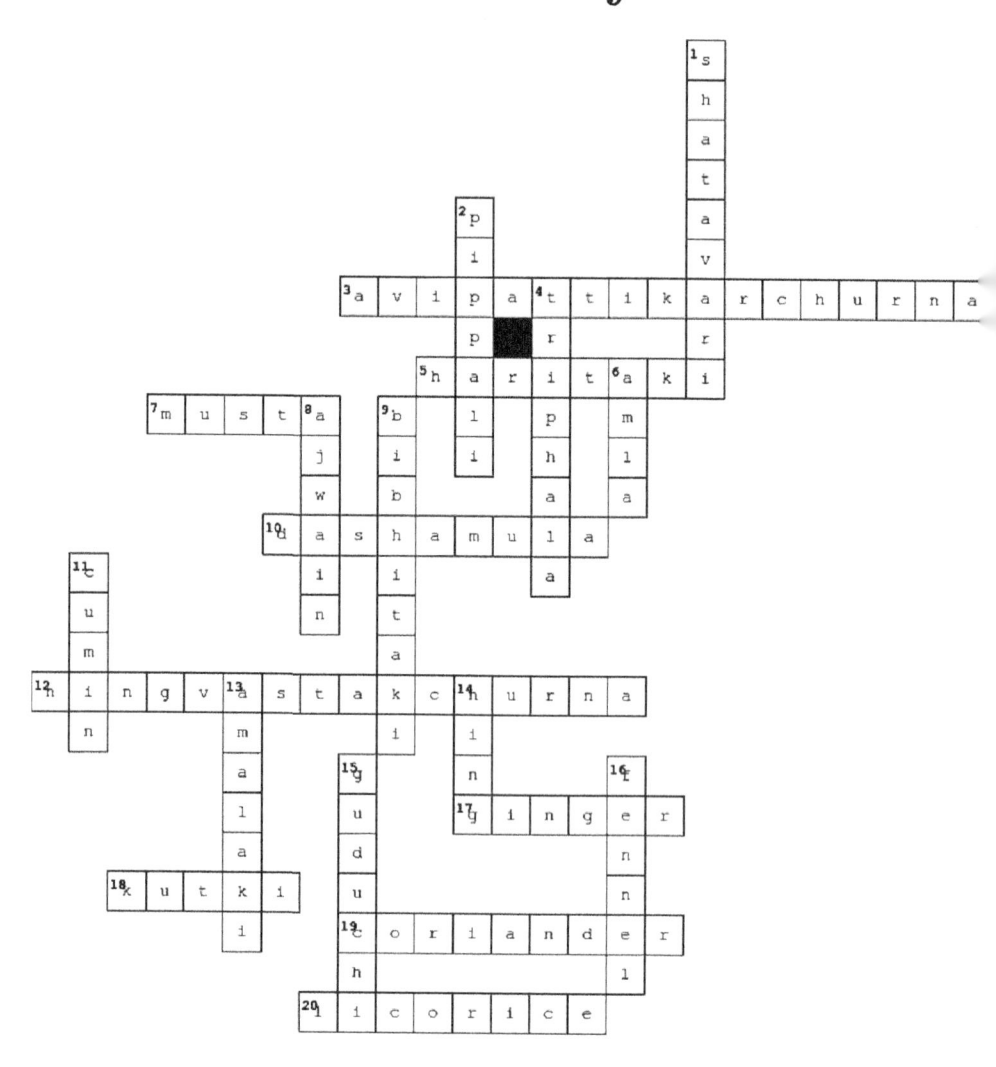

**Across:**
3. avipattikarchurna
5. haritaki
7. must
10. ashamula
12. ingva
14. churna
17. ginger
18. kuti
19. coriander
20. licorice

**Down:**
1. shatavara
2. pippali
4. trikatu
6. aki
8. ajwain
9. bibhitaki
11. cumin
13. amala
14. hing
15. gudu
16. fennel
19. ceh

82

Chapter 3

# Herbs for the Musculoskeletal System Answer Key

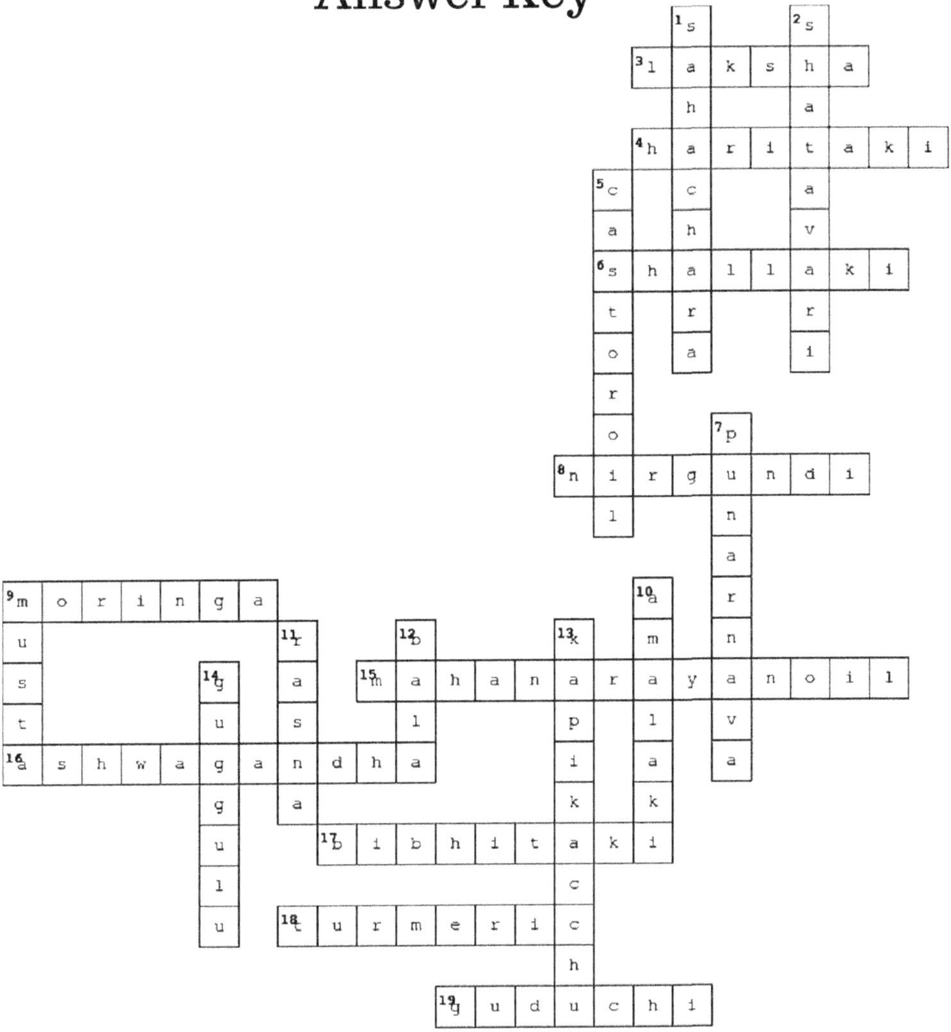

1 sahachara
2 shatavari
3 laksha
4 haritaki
5 castoroil
6 shallaki
7 punarnava
8 nirgundi
9 moringa
9 musta
10 amalaki
11 rasna
12 bala
13 kapikacchu
14 guggulu
15 mahanarayanoil
16 ashwagandha
17 bibhitaki
18 turmeric
19 guduchi

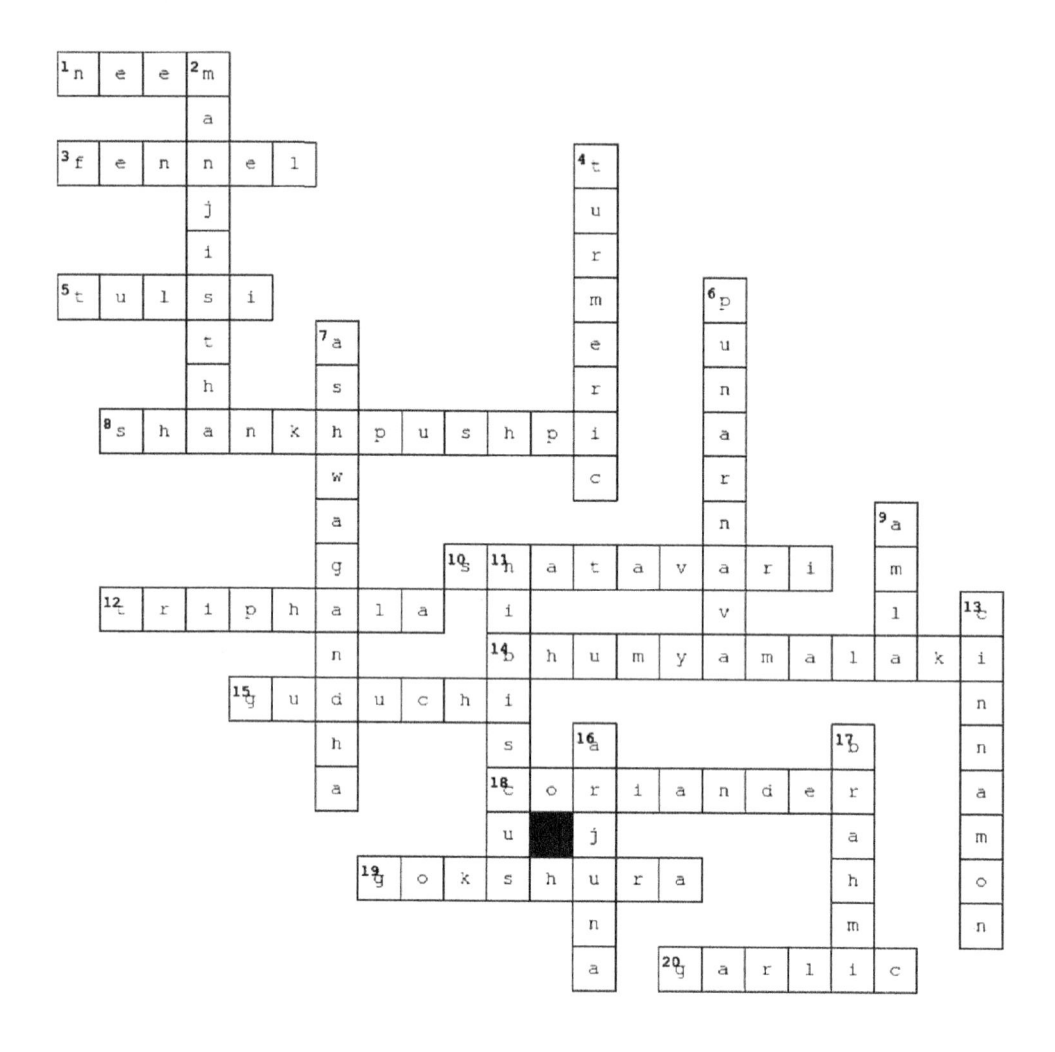

# Chapter 4
## Herbs for the Cardiovascular/Renal System Answer Key

**Across:**
1. neem
3. fennel
5. tulsi
8. shankhpushpi
11. atavari
12. triphala
14. humyamala
15. guduchi
18. coriander
19. gokshura
20. garlic

**Down:**
2. manjistha
4. turmeric
6. punarnava
7. ashwagandha
9. amla
10. shilajit
13. cinnamon
16. arjuna
17. brahmi

84

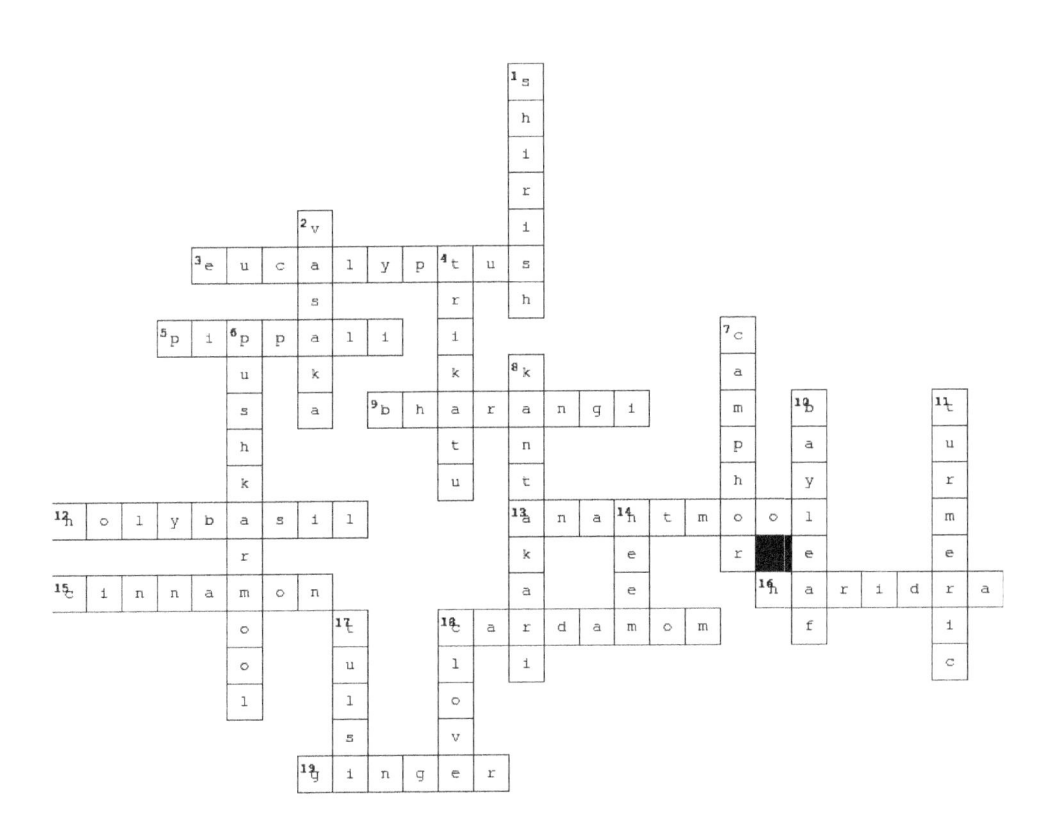

# Chapter 5
# Herbs for the Respiratory System Answer Key

# Chapter 6
# Herbs for the Articular System Answer Key

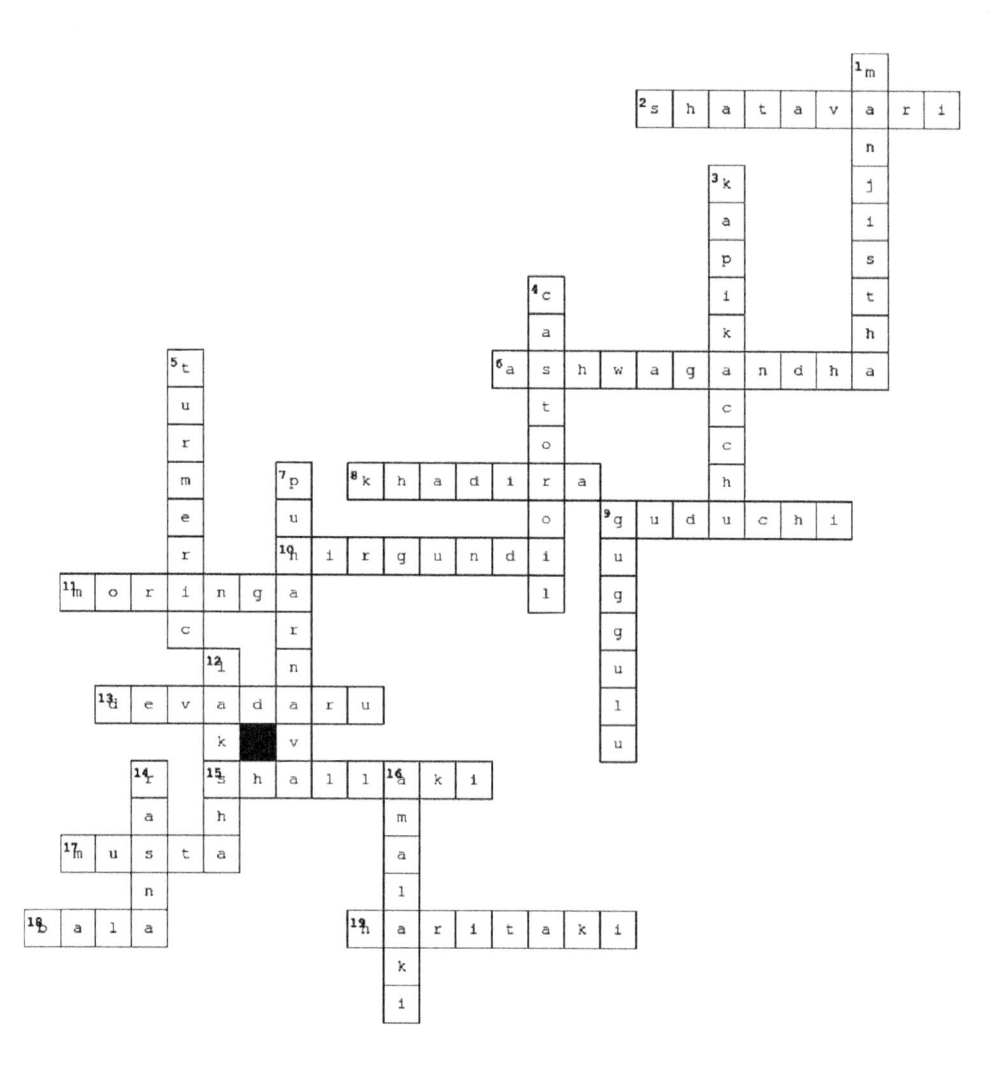

Across:
2. shatavari
6. ashwagandha
8. khadira
9. guduchi
10. nirgundi
11. moringa
13. devadaru
15. challa (shalli)
17. musta
18. bala
19. haritaki

Down:
1. manjistha
3. kapikacchu
4. catoli (catoru/ catoll)
5. turmeric
7. punarnava
9. guggulu
12. lina (? )
14. rasna
15. shank
16. amala

Grid letters (as shown):
- 1 down: m-a-n-j-i-s-t-h-a
- 2 across: s-h-a-t-a-v-a-r-i
- 3 down: k-a-p-i-k
- 4 down: c-a-t-o
- 5 down: t-u-r-m-e-r
- 6 across: a-s-h-w-a-g-a-n-d-h-a
- 7 down: p-u-u
- 8 across: k-h-a-d-i-r-a
- 9 across: g-u-d-u-c-h-i
- 9 down: g-u-g-g-u-l-u
- 10 across: n-i-r-g-u-n-d-i
- 11 across: m-o-r-i-n-g-a
- 12 down: l-i-n
- 13 across: d-e-v-a-d-a-r-u
- 14 down: r-a-n
- 15 across: h-a-l-l
- 15 down: s-h-h
- 16 down: a-m-a-l
- 17 across: m-u-s-t-a
- 18 across: b-a-l-a
- 19 across: h-a-r-i-t-a-k-i

86

# Chapter 7
## Herbs for the Endocrine/Reproductive System
## Answer Key

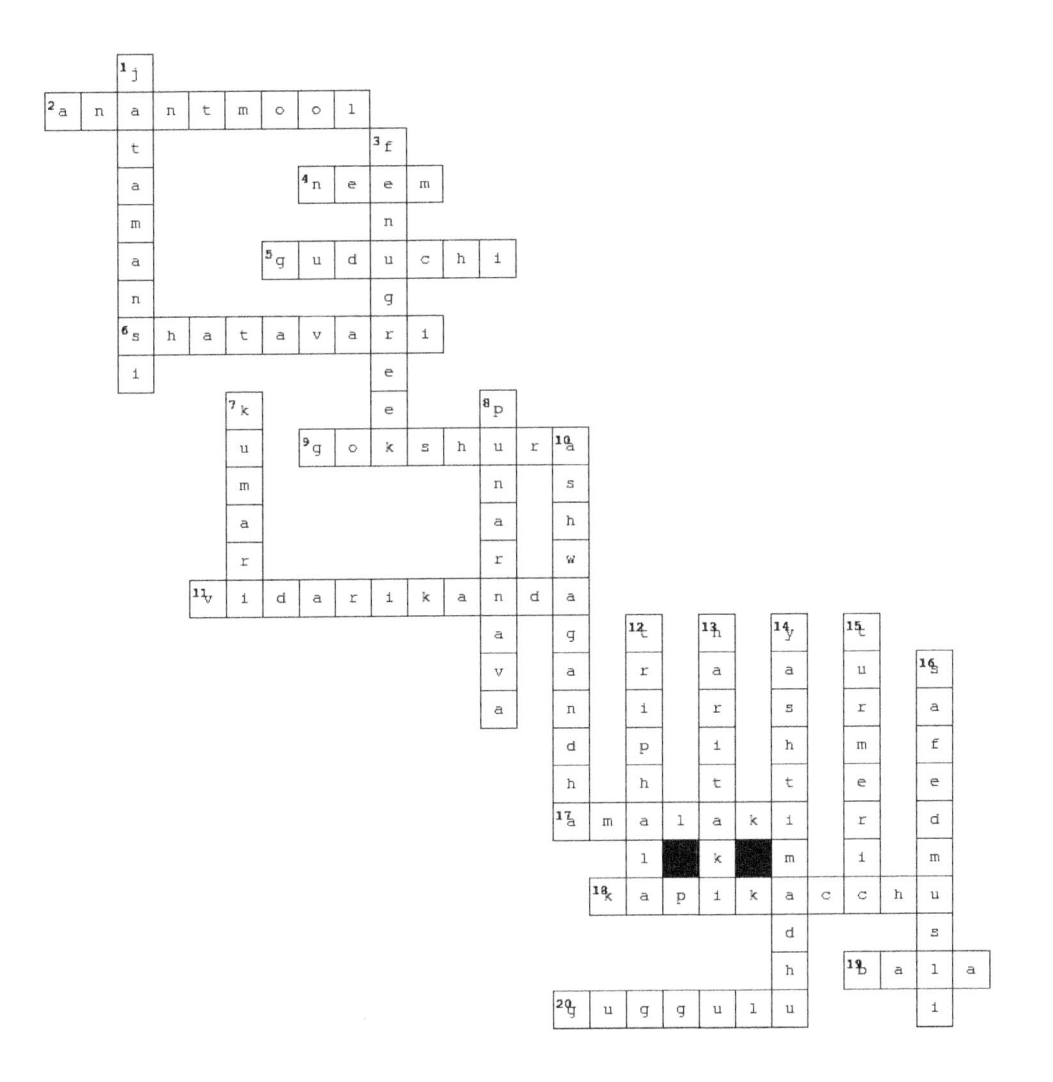

**Across:**
2. anantmool
4. neem
5. guduchi
6. shatavari
9. gokshur
11. vidarikand
17. amalaki
18. kapikacchu
19. bala
20. guggulu

**Down:**
1. j
3. fenugreek
7. kumari
8. punarvava (punarnava)
10. ashwagandha
12. tripalhi (tripraidh)
13. haripith
14. yashti
15. turmeri (turmeric)
16. safed

87

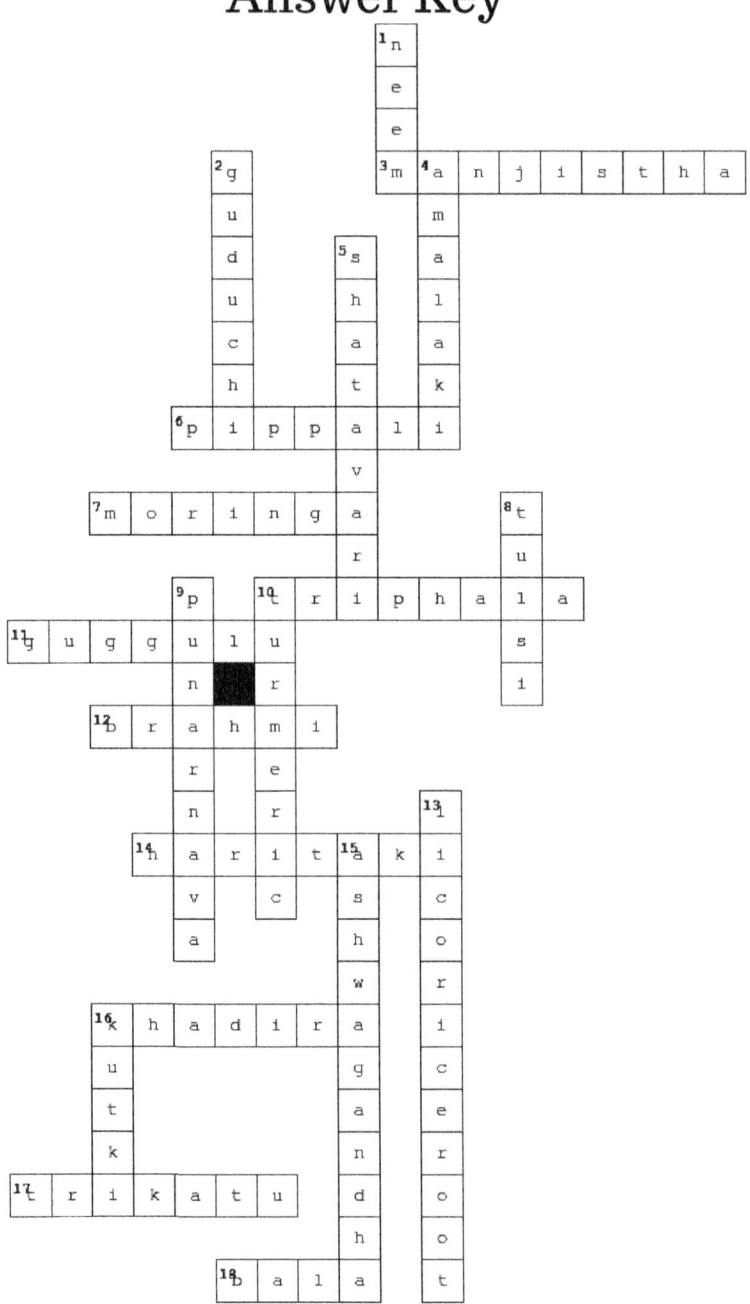

# Chapter 8
# Herbs for the Hematologic/Immunologic System Answer Key

|   |   |   |   |   |   |   |   | ¹n |   |   |   |   |   |   |   |
|---|---|---|---|---|---|---|---|----|---|---|---|---|---|---|---|
|   |   |   |   |   |   |   |   | e  |   |   |   |   |   |   |   |
|   |   |   |   |   |   |   |   | e  |   |   |   |   |   |   |   |
|   |   |   | ²g |   |   |   |   | ³m | ⁴a | n | j | i | s | t | h | a |
|   |   |   | u  |   |   |   |   |    | m  |   |   |   |   |   |   |
|   |   |   | d  |   |   | ⁵s |   |    | a  |   |   |   |   |   |   |
|   |   |   | u  |   |   | h  |   |    | l  |   |   |   |   |   |   |
|   |   |   | c  |   |   | a  |   |    | a  |   |   |   |   |   |   |
|   |   |   | h  |   |   | t  |   |    | k  |   |   |   |   |   |   |
|   |   | ⁶p | i  | p | p | a  | l | i  |    |   |   |   |   |   |   |
|   |   |    |    |   |   | v  |   |    |    |   |   |   |   |   |   |
|   | ⁷m | o | r | i | n | g  | a |    | ⁸t |   |   |   |   |   |   |
|   |    |   |   |   |   | r  |   |    | u  |   |   |   |   |   |   |
|   |    | ⁹p | ¹⁰t | r | i | p | h | a  | l  | a |   |   |   |   |   |
| ¹¹y | u | g | g | u | l | u  |   |    | s  |   |   |   |   |   |   |
|   |    |   | n |   | r |    |   |    | i  |   |   |   |   |   |   |
|   |    | ¹²b | r | a | h | m  | i |    |    |   |   |   |   |   |   |
|   |    |    | r |   | e |    |   |    |    |   |   |   |   |   |   |
|   |    |    | n |   | r |    |   | ¹³l |    |   |   |   |   |   |   |
|   |    | ¹⁴h | a | r | i | t  | ¹⁵a | k | i |   |   |   |   |   |
|   |    |    | v |   |   | c  | s |    | c  |   |   |   |   |   |   |
|   |    |    | a |   |   |    | h |    | o  |   |   |   |   |   |   |
|   |    |    |   |   |   |    | w |    | r  |   |   |   |   |   |   |
|   |    | ¹⁶k | h | a | d | i  | r | a  | i  |   |   |   |   |   |   |
|   |    | u  |   |   |   |    | g |    | c  |   |   |   |   |   |   |
|   |    | t  |   |   |   |    | a |    | e  |   |   |   |   |   |   |
|   |    | k  |   |   |   |    | n |    | r  |   |   |   |   |   |   |
| ¹⁷t | r | i | k | a | t | u  | d |    | o  |   |   |   |   |   |   |
|   |    |    |   |   |   |    | h |    | o  |   |   |   |   |   |   |
|   |    |    |   |   | ¹⁸b | a | l | a  | t  |   |   |   |   |   |   |

# Chapter 9
## Herbs for the Skin
## Answer Key

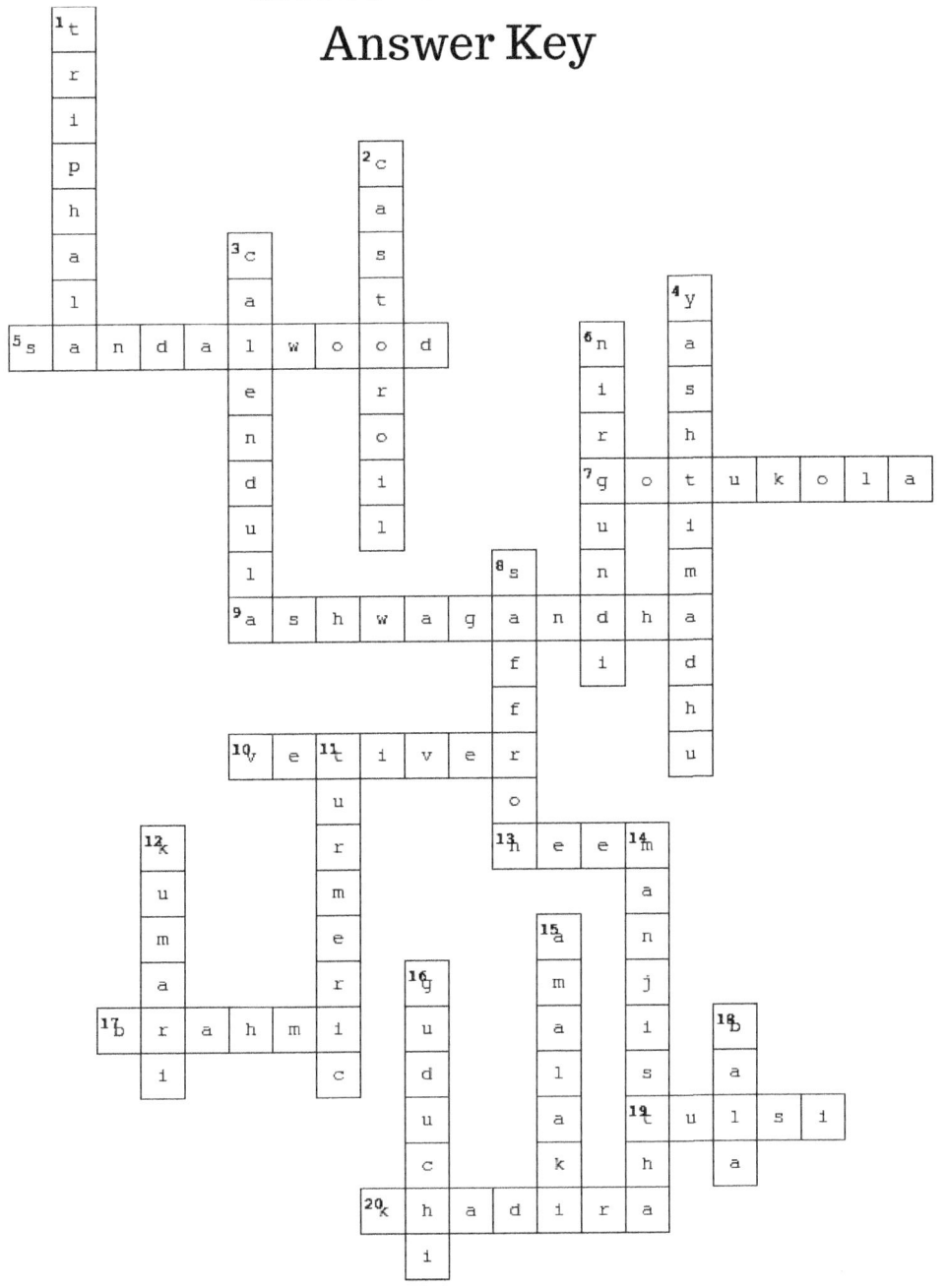

**Across:**
5. sandalwood
7. gotukola
9. ashwaganda
10. vetiver
13. hee (neem area)
17. brahmi
19. tulsi
20. khadira

**Down:**
1. triphala
2. castor
3. calendula
4. yashu...
6. nirgundi
8. saffron
11. turmeric
12. kumari
14. manjistha
15. amalaki
16. guduchi
18. ba...

89

# Chapter 10
# Herbs for the Nervous System Answer Key

**Across:**
1. turmeric
3. gotukola
4. liceroot
6. shatavari
9. anantmool
11. kava
12. kava
13. agar
15. hutmeg
16. tulsi

**Down:**
2. mucunaprurien
5. pippali
7. maduk
8. vacha
10. jyoshimahami
11. kaprari
12. kalilisu
14. guggu

# Chapter 11
# Herbs that Detoxify
# Answer Key

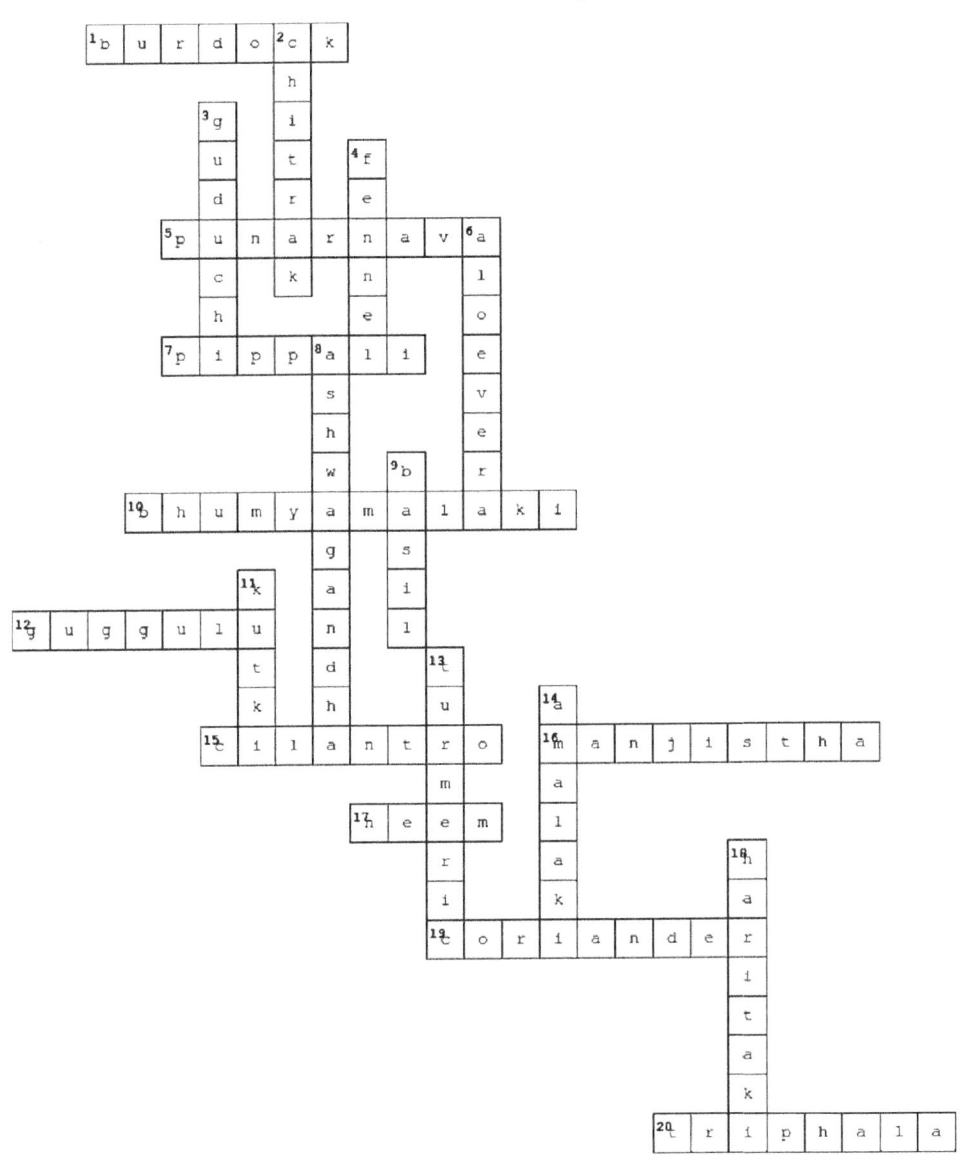

Across:
1. burdock
5. punarnava
7. pippali
10. bhumyamalaki
12. guggulu
15. cilantro
16. manjistha
17. neem
19. coriander
20. triphala

Down:
2. chitrak
3. gudduchi
4. fenugreek
6. aloevera
8. ashwagandha
9. bsri (brahmi)
11. kaṭuki
13. tumari (turmeric)
14. alaka
18. haritaki

91

# Chapter 12
# Herbs for Emotional/Mental Well-being Answer Key

**Across:**
6. valerian
10. holy basil
13. rhodiola
14. gotu kola
15. lemon balm
16. jatamansi
17. passionflower
20. rosemary

**Down:**
1. peppermint
2. kavakava
3. brahmi
4. lemon verbena
5. ginkgo biloba
7. saffron
8. hemp
9. skullcap
11. chamomile
12. lavender
18. skullcap
19. ashwagandha

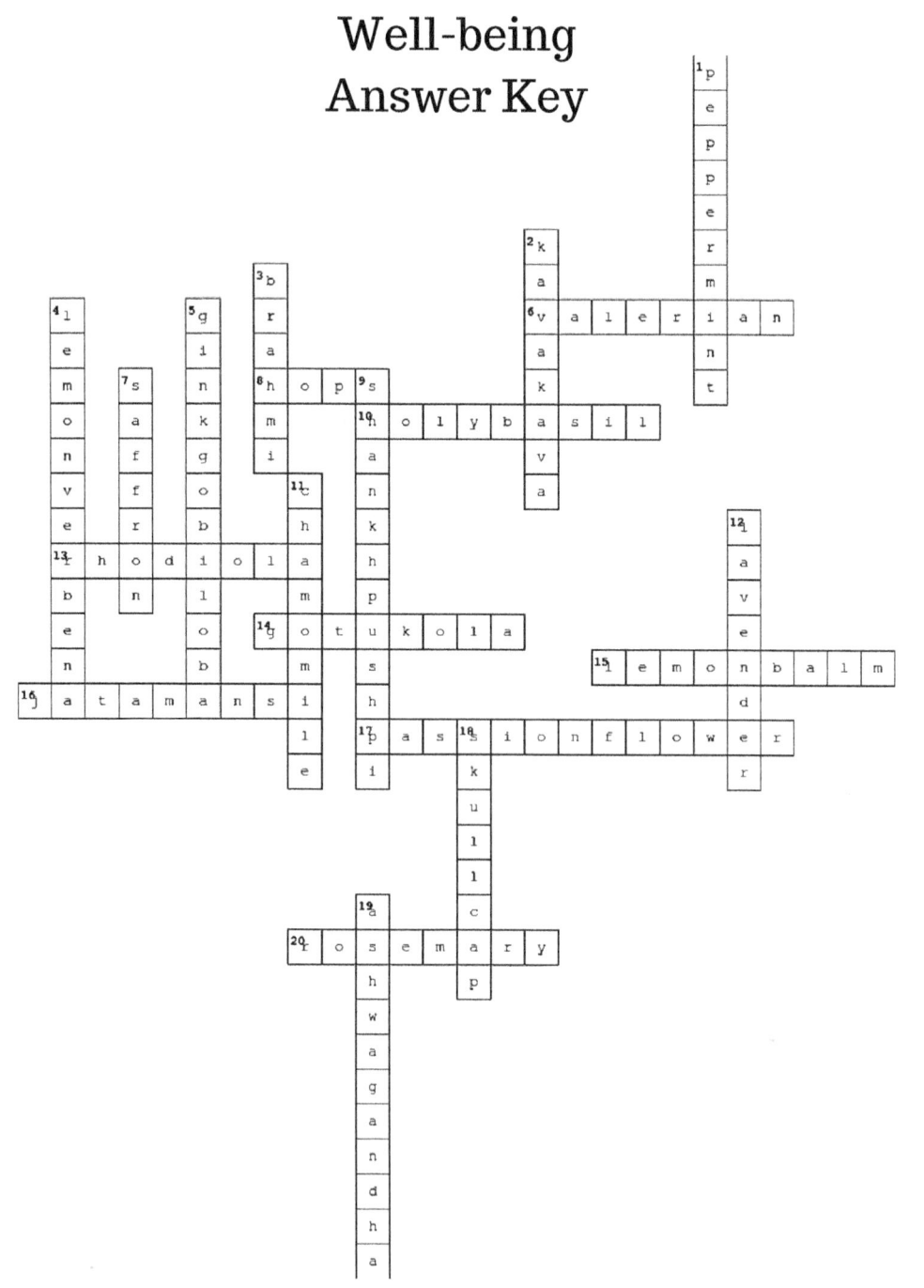

# About the Authors

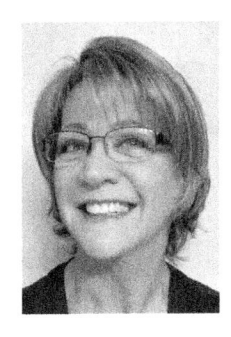

Carol Paredes transitioned from a successful 30-year career in technology to a dedication to health and wellness. She graduated summa cum laude with a B.S. in Software Development. Now, as an Ayurvedic Practitioner, Certified Integrative Nutrition Health Coach, and Yoga instructor, Carol shares her expertise in Maryland and Delaware.

In March 2020, Carol joined the Physiology and Health Department at Maharishi International University, earning her M.S. in Maharishi AyurVeda and Integrative Medicine by June 2020. She currently serves as Associate Chair of the department, blending her knowledge in technology and wellness to guide others towards holistic living and self-discovery. Carol's unique perspective and dedication make her a beacon of wisdom and empowerment in promoting holistic well-being.

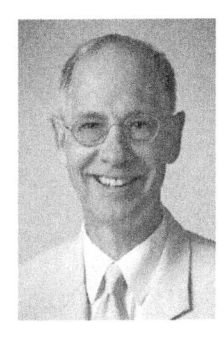

Dr. Robert Keith Wallace completed pioneering research on the Transcendental Meditation technique. His seminal papers on a fourth major state of consciousness-published in Science, American Journal of Physiology, and Scientific American-support a new paradigm of mind-body medicine and total brain development.

Dr. Wallace was the founding President of Maharishi International University and has traveled around the world giving lectures at major universities and institutes, and has written and co-authored several books. He is presently a Trustee of Maharishi International University and Chairman of the Department of Physiology and Health.

Printed in Great Britain
by Amazon